Not the Worst Thing

Life and Death in Clinical Ethics

Leslie Beckhart Jenal
with Jesse Moreno

Instructor's Guide Available

For Instructors:

I will send you my complete course, including supplemental reading, quizzes (mostly true/false and short answer), film recommendations, video clips, and all other resources that I have used for this course. The materials will be sent to you on a USB drive.

Please write me a letter on your institution's letterhead, scan the signed letter, and email it to me at lkbj@jjenal.com.

A shipping fee of $10.00 will be charged.

To my husband, Jim, and my daughter, Julia, who have heard me struggle with the material in the book –

and encouraged me to write rather than making them listen to me anymore.

CONTENTS

Preface

I have written this book because I have compassion for patients and their loved ones. The Latin root *pati*, meaning to suffer, is the root of the words *patient* - the one who suffers - and *compassion* - the response to the suffering of others. In all my years as an ethicist at medical centers, as a hospital chaplain working in intensive care units and later as a hospice chaplain, I have suffered with the suffering of patients and their loved ones.

I have also taught clinical ethics to hundreds of nursing students for over a decade. This book is based on my lecture notes, case studies, and experience. I am deeply indebted to these students. It has been a joy and an honor to watch them progress from believing that biological life must be preserved at all costs, to a greater compassion for the suffering of a patient receiving aggressive treatment for no good reason. I hope that I teach my students about human life and the love of life. And when biological life can be let go.

I am also deeply grateful to my husband and my daughter, who have heard me explore and be saddened by these topics for more years than I can count. This book is dedicated to them: Jim and Julia.

Introduction

Death is *not* the worst thing. Death is inevitable. At some point, we are all going to be beyond medical rescue.

A bad death *is* the worst thing that can happen.

A natural death, at home among loved ones, with pain and other symptoms well managed, can be blessed and meaningful–*as well* as inevitable. A death in an intensive care unit, plugged into a mechanical ventilator, with tubes and pumps in every orifice (some natural and some manufactured), dying with broken ribs and burned skin after forty minutes of cardiopulmonary resuscitation is mercifully ended–*that* is the worst thing.

There is a vast difference between biological life (the life of the body alone) and the lives that we want to live. Medicine is capable of supporting a life with *quality*. Medicine is also capable of destroying a human life in the interests of saving a body. Medicine can be both a blessing and a curse.

We will start with a consideration of the quality of a human life: what we are willing to live with and when we are willing to let go. We will then explore ordinary medical treatment, that we *should* provide, and extraordinary treatment, which we *may* provide. We will discuss how a patient makes an informed choice about treatment, when that patient has the capacity to make a decision, and who makes the decision for the patient when she cannot do so for herself. We will discuss futile treatment, which we must never provide, and how to address conflicts between healthcare providers who refuse it and loved ones who demand it. We will look at the relationship between rationing end-of-life treatments and kind end-of-life treatment. We will discover what to do when all else fails, namely: palliative sedation, aggressive pain management, stopping eating and drinking, and physician-assisted suicide and euthanasia.

I hope that everything in this book is grounded in the suffering of the patient and our compassionate response to her. Let us begin with what it means to have a human life and how we might stay human after all the medical treatment ends.

Chapter 1. Quality of Life

Case 1-1. An End-Stage Dementia Patient and Cardiopulmonary Resuscitation.

Herbert Jones is eighty years old and lives in a skilled nursing facility. He has end-stage dementia and is at this point cognitively vegetative and unaware of his surroundings or of other people. However, his family has directed that the television be left on twenty-four hours a day. Herbert is fed by a percutaneous endoscopic gastrostomy (PEG) tube in his abdomen (a surgically placed feeding tube pumping nutrients directly into his stomach). He has a catheter to collect his urine and must wear a diaper because he is incontinent of bowel movements.

Herbert is severely contracted. His feet are folded up and crossed adjacent to his buttocks; his arms are crossed over his chest. He has decubitus ulcers (deep tissue wounds) because of the contractures. As a result, Herbert has undergone several surgical amputations. He lost his right foot and all the toes on his left foot. Herbert has been admitted to the hospital numerous times due to aspiration pneumonia, wherein the feedings have gone directly into his lungs and caused infections. His four children demand that he be treated with antibiotics every time aspiration occurs. Herbert is a full code, meaning that his family is demanding cardiopulmonary resuscitation (CPR) in the event that he stops breathing and his heart stops.

One evening, Herbert suddenly stops breathing. His heart stops shortly thereafter. The paramedics should break Herbert's arms to get at his chest in order to perform the chest compressions entailed by cardiopulmonary resuscitation. Herbert is resuscitated after fifteen minutes and is sent to the emergency room of a local hospital with two badly broken arms and several broken ribs. His family demands admission to the intensive care unit.

Discussion Questions

- Before reading the remainder of the chapter, what in your opinion is Herbert's quality of life?
- Would you want to continue to be alive if you had Herbert's quality of life?
- Does Herbert's medical treatment enhance his quality of life?
- Does Herbert's medical treatment worsen his quality of life?

If we believe that we will die, sometime and somehow at some point, and hope that our death will be meaningful and comfortable, we already know that biological life is not the ultimate value. We already know that our biological life should not be preserved at all costs. The duty to preserve biological life is not absolute—we must recognize a limit.

Most bioethicists use the term *biological life* to reference the patient's physical body alone while the term *human life* defines the entirety of the patient—including the body but also includes the intellectual, emotional, and existential meaning of the patient's total self.

We may use the term *quality of life* to ground our beliefs. *Quality of life* will define the borders of the otherwise absolute value of biological life. Quality of life considerations will often—and should—circumscribe our duty to sustain purely biological life. Without an adequate concept of quality of life, we will be forced to extract every possible moment of biological life from a patient, condemning the patient and his family and friends to suffering and pain far beyond their capacity to bear it, or indeed, the need.

Some bioethicists have proposed a distinction between a *human being* and a *human person*. This distinction means, whether they admit it or not, that decisions should be made based upon the instrumental and social value of a life. When we distinguish between a human being and a human person, the necessary inference is that some human beings are non-persons. Patients who lack the potential for cognitive ability are the first to fall into this category. Severely developmentally disabled patients, end-stage dementia patients, permanently unconscious patients, and patients with severe traumatic brain injuries, for example, would not be considered complete persons under this distinction. The argument is that we owe nothing to a patient who is not a person, that a non-personal life is not worth living. The blanket distinction between a human being and a human person has been used to justify genocide and the forced sterilization of the developmentally disabled and so we must be highly wary of wide-based generalizations.

For other bioethicists, a patient has no *quality of life* if he lacks the capacity for human relationship and its fundamental prerequisite—self-awareness. Specifically, the contention is that a patient has quality of life only when he has observable neocortical function. The idea is that some criteria, properties, attributes, or categories must be present before we can determine that the patient has an appreciable quality of life. These objective criteria are facts determined by those who have responsibility for the patient. If these criteria are absent, then we do not have responsibility for a patient; we have responsibility for an object. This life has no social and functional utility. The patient cannot *do* anything. The argument is that the patient merely exists, and existence is not enough.

In this book, we are not rejecting all quality of life determinations; we are rejecting quality of life determinations made by people other than the patient and based on the properties, attributes, and categories of the patient's life. However, the real issue is that only the *patient* can judge whether his or her life is worth living. Unfortunately, quality of life judgments can easily be interpreted as a code for those inclined toward judging a life as worthless.

Nevertheless, we *do* have an intuition or belief that the values of self-awareness and the capacity for human relationship are essential to human life. *The values of self-awareness and the capacity for human relationships are at the heart of our own lives.* Most of us would not want to live in a state where these two values, or the potential to enjoy these two values, are wholly absent. This is not to say that the lives of patients who do not have at least the *potential* for self-awareness and human relationship are worthless. We also have the intuition that all biological lives have equal value and genuinely incalculable worth. However, whether a life is worth living is for the patient to determine—no other. Again, quality of life should never be determined merely by the relative values of lives in contrast. At its core, this becomes an argument of self-determination.

If at least the potential to be self-aware and to enjoy human relationships is at the core of our being, then an understanding of a quality of life is determined by those virtues. In addition, there are other values that anyone might consider essential to their lives, such as:

- Our cognitive abilities and the ability to exercise our intelligence.

- The capacity to contribute in a meaningful way to society.

- Our capacity for self-determination.

- Our independence.

Pursuing these values (and others) gives our lives quality. If we can pursue our life's values, we have a quality of life. When we can pursue our life's values, then our lives feel worth living.

Consider a few examples:

- A sixty-year-old mathematics professor refuses to take a cardiac medication because it is associated with a higher risk of dementia. He would rather die of a heart attack than risk losing his cognition and self-awareness.

- A thirty-three-year-old woman with uterine cancer chooses to use an experimental chemotherapy that causes chemical burns inside her esophagus in the hopes that she will have more time with her young children.

- An eighty-five-year-old man chooses to have quadruple bypass and mitral valve replacement in his heart because it offers him the chance to continue to play golf every day.

- A thirty-three-year-old divorced man with Amyotrophic Lateral Sclerosis (ALS) chooses to live his last days in a nursing home rather than feeling like a burden to his elderly mother.

We are not advocating the sanctity of biological life ethic, also known as a vitalist ethic. When we believe that biological life is a higher value than self-awareness, then biological life must be preserved at all costs—even that of immense pain and suffering. Biological life has value, just as health and consciousness have value. However, the meaning of the patient's whole, human life is the ultimate and absolute value. *Biological life is an instrumental good, not an absolute value*. To argue otherwise is to reduce all of human existence to the physical body. The sanctity-of-life position disregards "values about life and the way it should be lived."[1] We are advocating the promotion of the *purpose and meaning* of a biological life. Quality of life includes the value of biological life but goes beyond it. Biological life can be let go.

Patients make quality of life determinations all the time based on their perceptions of what makes life worth living. Patients consider (and often under these circumstances, discover) their core values, such as their ability to tolerate pain or the perceived indignity of being helpless and dependent on others. Patients may choose to avoid being a burden to family and friends. At some point, most patients are willing to let their biological lives go.

The goal of any medical treatment must be to promote the patient's quality of life. Medical treatment should not frustrate, impede, or eliminate the patient's quality of life. When medical treatment will frustrate or even eliminate the patient's quality of life, then medicine has reached the end of its own reason for existence.[2]

This means that the patient's quality of life is based on a relationship. The patient's perceived quality of life, centered on him or herself, is not of itself enough to determine whether a medical treatment should be provided or foregone. The patient's medical condition must promote that patient's quality of life. The patient makes a subjective and evaluative judgment about his or her quality of life. However, the relationship between the patient's ability to enjoy that quality of life and the patient's medical condition is objective. It is a simple fact that one way or the other a medical treatment will promote or frustrate the patient's quality of life. Quality of life takes into account the value of the treatment to the patient, along with whatever suffering that it entails. Medical treatment must always be focused on the relationship of the patient's medical condition to his or her quality of life.[3] Medicine should have a heart.

Death need not always be resisted at the cost of immense suffering, as if absolutely everything is an improvement over death.[4] Pure biological life is not of incalculable worth. Rather, human lives are of incalculable worth. Human life, with all the existential, intellectual, spiritual, emotional, and physical values that it enables, is of ultimate value. Biological life need not be, and should not be, preserved at all costs. Pursuing the truths of all that is meant by "quality of life" is a search for what makes life worth living - what it is *not* is some crude conviction that the values of lives are relative.

Case 1-2. A Critically Ill Patient and the Activities That Make Life Worth Living.

Seventy-five-year-old Edna Lingstrom has a major cardiac arrest while undergoing a cardiac catheterization, a diagnostic procedure following her heart attack the day before. The cardiac team performs cardiopulmonary resuscitation (CPR) all the way to the operating room. The cardiothoracic surgeon who is to perform the operation on Edna's failing heart approaches her husband, Joe, in the waiting room, to get consent for the surgery. There is no time for Joe to think when he is confronted by this emergency. He gives consent immediately and automatically, and the surgery goes forward.

For the first week, Edna remains ventilator-dependent in the intensive care unit (ICU). She is sedated. When the sedation wears off, she is delirious. Joe is constantly at Edna's bedside. Joe begins to realize that Edna, if she survives, will require an extended recovery period. Joe also has failing health and would be unable to care for Edna during her recovery. Joe realizes that if Edna survives, she would have to be placed in a rehabilitation facility or in a skilled nursing facility (a nursing home) for some time before coming home, if she ever comes home.

The Lingstroms had filled out advance directives when they made their living trust. They each named the other to make decisions. They had also extensively discussed what medical interventions they did and did not want. The advance directives evidenced the content of these discussions. Ed now believes that he had consented to the cardiac surgery without understanding the extensive recovery period resulting from the surgery. In Edna's advance directive, she had explicitly stated that she would not want to be placed in either a rehabilitation facility or in a skilled nursing facility. Edna stated in her advance directive that she wanted to die at home. Yet Joe's failing health would make caring for Edna impossible. There is no money for private caregivers, but the couple would qualify for Medicaid, which would pay for a skilled nursing facility.

Joe now feels that he had betrayed Edna by consenting to the cardiac surgery now that he sees the long recovery period that it would entail. He knows that Edna is a very active woman and values her independence. Many times, she had stated what she did not want: "To be kept alive on machines. That's no life." Subsequent to Edna's retirement from her work as an accountant, she had played tennis every day. She had even joked that tennis was what made her life worth living. Joe had been hurt by this statement at the time, but now he understood Edna's meaning.

However, the surgeon and the cardiologist do not think that Edna's long recovery period is unreasonable. When Joe requests a Do-Not-Resuscitate (DNR) order and begins talking to the nurses about discontinuing aggressive treatment, the surgeon contacts the medical center's ethics committee.

The ethics consultants speak with all parties involved and hear their views. They speak to the surgeon, the cardiologist, two of Edna's nurses in the ICU, the medical social worker, and the ICU chaplain. They also speak to Joe. When Edna is awake, she is not alert, and the ethics consultants cannot communicate with her. Joe is very emotional. He feels that he failed Edna now he sees what her treatment entails. The surgeon and the cardiologist are made uncomfortable by Joe's emotion. Joe repeatedly and tearfully maintains that Edna did not want to be kept alive on machines. Now, she is dependent on a ventilator to breathe.

The cardiologist explains that Edna is not expected to become permanently ventilator-dependent. However, when Joe presses him, he acknowledges that the ventilator settings would have to be lowered bit-by-bit over several days, and there is always the chance that Edna would experience respiratory distress and require ventilator support again. The surgeon is optimistic that Edna could be successfully weaned from the ventilator and would make a complete recovery, given time and treatment. He is unwilling to speculate as to how much time Edna would need to recover. Although the surgeon opposes any limitations on life-sustaining treatment, he does agree to a Do-Not-Resuscitate (DNR) order specifying that if Edna's heart fails, no chest compressions would be done.

Edna's weaning process is very slow and a tracheostomy has to be performed. Edna is no longer receiving ventilator support from a tube down her throat. Now, the ventilator is inserted into a surgically made hole in her throat. She is also found to have sepsis, a major life-threatening systemic infection. Joe begins to realize that even if Edna survives, her recovery would be uncertain and long, longer than Edna would tolerate if she were able to speak her mind. Joe knows that even if Edna survives, her extensive recovery would be unacceptable to her. Now, Joe wants to stop all medical treatment, including the ventilator, despite the surgeon's belief that Edna could be weaned. Joe also regrets his earlier consent to a feeding tube to support Edna's body with nutrients while she recovered.

Specifically, Edna had stated in her advance directive that tube feeding could be provided if she had a chance for a full recovery. The advance directive also stated that any artificial feeding should be stopped if it became clear that she would suffer physical or mental disability at a level that was unacceptable to her. Under the terms of Edna's advance directive, Joe has the right to make all medical decisions for Edna. The surgeon and the cardiologist medical team do not want him to demand that the feedings be stopped. They feel that Edna still has a chance for a meaningful recovery, given time and extensive medical treatment. The surgeon in particular maintains his optimism. He believes that Edna's advance directive implies that she would accept a feeding tube during her recovery. On the other hand, the social worker and the chaplain understand that Edna might not have a full recovery and might be left in a state in which she would not want to live, just as Joe was saying.

After a family meeting, a compromise was reached. No further treatments would be added but the ventilator and feeding tube would not be stopped. Over the next two days, Edna's infection becomes overwhelming. The surgeon finally admits that Edna's prognosis now is very poor. The intensivist (the ICU physician) remove the ventilator and clamps the feeding tube. She also directs that opiates be given to Edna so that she will not suffer from air hunger when the ventilator is removed. Two hours after the ventilator is withdrawn, Edna dies in Joe's arms.

Discussion Questions

- Knowing what you know about Edna, what is the minimum quality of life with which she would be willing to live? Do you believe that Edna would accept a feeding tube during a long and uncertain recovery?

- What if Edna would not make a full recovery? Suppose she were in a wheelchair permanently?

- If Edna would be in a wheelchair, Joe's health would limit how much care he could provide to her. What if Edna ended up in a skilled nursing facility permanently? Would she be willing to live this way?

- How many weeks or months would you be willing to accept extensive medical treatment, including a tracheostomy and a feeding tube, if your recovery would be uncertain?

Case 1-3. A Mother and a Child.

Her physicians inform a young woman, Jai, in her eighth month of pregnancy, that she has lung cancer. She delivers the baby at thirty-six weeks by caesarean section. The next day, Jai undergoes a first round of chemotherapy. After two weeks, it is determined that her cancer cells do not have the genetic mutation that the chemotherapy targets. She starts a second round of chemotherapy. Her cancer metastasizes and spreads to other organs. She undergoes a third round of chemotherapy while her oncologists frantically search for an experimental drug that might prolong her life.

The second and third rounds of chemotherapy cause severe symptoms. Her hands and feet are numb. She has so much fluid in her belly that her breathing is impaired. A technician repeatedly removes the fluid but, as fast as it is removed, it comes back. Jai loses forty pounds because she is so nauseous and vomiting so frequently that she cannot keep any food down. Jai is more comfortable when she does not eat or drink.

The third round of chemotherapy impairs Jai's immune system so drastically that her baby must be kept away from her whenever he has a cough or the sniffles. As Jai's cancer spreads, not holding the baby because the baby is sick has become irrelevant. Jai is now so weak that she cannot support the baby in her arms even when she is lying down. One day, she cannot breathe. She is rushed to the hospital and put on a ventilator. Her family finally realizes that Jai is dying and asks that the ventilator be withdrawn.

Discussion Questions

- Does Jai's cancer treatment affect her ability to pursue the values that make her life worth living? Specifically, does the fact that she cannot hold her baby mean that her quality of life is impaired?

- Would you be willing to undergo a third round of chemotherapy for the uncertain chance that it would prolong your life without curing your cancer?

- Would you take an experimental drug with unknown side effects if it would prolong your life for three weeks in Jai's condition?

Chapter 2. Killing versus Allowing to Die

Case 2-1. Dementia and Artificial Nutrition and Hydration.

James Ardis, a widowed, incontinent ninety-two-year-old man, is brought to the emergency room of a community hospital in respiratory distress due to aspiration pneumonia. While in the emergency room, he is found to have a urinary tract infection. James lives with his daughter Olivia, her husband, her two adult children, and Olivia's three grandchildren. Eighteen months previously, James had begun to refuse food and fluids and had become lethargic and confused. A gastrostomy tube was placed for artificial nutrition and hydration. Now, James is extremely contracted. He had a stage four decubitus ulcer–down to the bone–on his coccyx and stage three ulcers of both elbows and heels. He is minimally responsive and reacts only to deeply painful stimuli. He neither grimaces nor calls out when he is repositioned or when his wounds are cleaned and redressed.

James is treated with antibiotics for the urinary tract infection and the pneumonia, and receives intravenous hydration. Artificial nutrition is continued. When James is awake, he stares at the wall. He does not respond to the nurses or to his family. After several days of antibiotics, artificial nutrition, and hydration, there is no improvement in his mental status and, finally, he is diagnosed with advanced dementia. Because James has no quality of life, his physicians question whether continued aggressive treatment is in James' best interests. Specifically, they question whether continued antibiotic treatment of the urinary tract infection and the pneumonia is compassionate. The physicians believe that a Do-Not-Resuscitate order should be written, the antibiotics should be withdrawn, the pneumonia should be allowed to take its course, and James' symptoms should be treated with oxygen, Tylenol, and morphine. In addition, they believe that the artificial nutrition should be withdrawn, as James will die of the pneumonia before he will die of starvation.

Discussion Questions

- What is James's quality of life? Can he pursue any values that might make his life worth living?

- Do you believe that it is unethical not to provide antibiotics that might cure James's pneumonia? Do we always need to provide antibiotics because they are so easy to provide?

- If James were to receive antibiotics and his pneumonia were cured, then have we taken away James's opportunity to die?

- Would you want to live with James's current quality of life?

- If James were to miraculously be able to communicate for five minutes, knowing that he would then lapse back into his condition, do you think he would want to continue to live this way?

- If we withhold the antibiotics, should we also withdraw his feeding tube and any intravenous hydration that he might be receiving? Is withdrawing the feeding tube murder?

Death in the hospital is no longer a *bona mors* (a good death), a carefully planned event following a religious ritual or the patient's carefully considered last words. Death in the hospital is a technical phenomenon and is frequently the result of the withdrawal or withholding of life-sustaining treatment. Ineffective and painful cardiopulmonary resuscitation often functions as *last rites*. Most of the time, the patient has already lost consciousness by the time life-sustaining treatment is withheld or withdrawn. Death in the hospital comes after a myriad of medical decisions, making it impossible to know at what point the patient irrevocably lost consciousness, or respiratory drive, or cardiac function. These little deaths precede the *final* death–the one in which the time of death is determined more by the physician's signature on a chart than by the patient's actual terminal process.

Medical treatments for dying patients include treatments intended to:

- Cure disease
- Prolong biological life with hope of recovery, especially hope of recovering consciousness
- Compensate for other treatments causing iatrogenic harm (side effects)
- Slow disease progression
- Compensate for a failure of an organ of the body
- Prolong biological life
- Prolong the dying process

Life-sustaining treatment, or life support, is any medical intervention that attempts to prolong biological life without reversing the underlying fatal pathology. A fatal pathology is any disease, illness, or injury that will cause death if untreated and allowed to run its course. A fatal pathology differs from a *terminal illness*, which is defined as an illness where the patient's death will probably occur within six months. The set of fatal pathologies includes the subset of terminal illnesses.

Legally and ethically, the decision to end life-sustaining treatment is made by the patient. The decision may also be made by a surrogate who is responsible for the patient.[1] When circumstances are such that further medical treatment will only prolong the patient's dying process, then allowing the patient to die by withdrawing or withholding life-sustaining treatment and providing appropriate comfort care is not only permissible, it is morally right and it is kind.

Life-sustaining treatment may be withheld (never started in the first place) or withdrawn (stopped after it has been started). If life-sustaining treatment is justifiably withheld or withdrawn, the ethical and legal cause of the patient's death is the underlying fatal pathology. When withholding or withdrawing life-sustaining treatment is justifiable, the ethical and legal cause of death is the underlying fatal pathology that caused the patient to receive the life-sustaining treatment in the first place. In other words, if a patient receives ventilator treatment because she overdosed on opiates and cannot breathe on her own, and if the ventilator is subsequently withdrawn, the patient's ethical and legal cause of death is the drug overdose. If a patient has head and brain trauma because of a motorcycle accident and cannot breathe, and subsequently the ventilator is withdrawn, the patient dies of the trauma from the motorcycle accident. The same goes for an end-stage dementia patient receiving artificially administered nutrients. When the feeding tube is withdrawn, the patient dies of end-stage dementia when the patient could not eat because she forgot how to swallow.

When life-sustaining treatment is justifiably withheld or withdrawn, death is foreseen but the patient is not killed. Withholding or withdrawing life-sustaining treatment may bring about death, but it is *not* killing.

There is a vast moral difference between killing a patient and *allowing a patient to die* (even in dying patients). Killing involves injury. Allowing to die involves non-benefit.[2] As medical professionals, we have a higher duty not to kill patients than the duty we have not to allow them to die—this is a vital distinction. In allowing a patient to die, we are not interfering with an inevitable death. We cease to prevent an ongoing, irrevocable, and natural process of dying. Is it not right to comply with a dying patient's voluntary and cognizant request to die by withholding or withdrawing life-sustaining treatment? The patient places no value on their continued life or believes that continued life will be burdensome, unbeneficial, and altogether miserable. The patient clearly believes that his or her continued life fails to promote (or even outright harms) the quality of life acceptable to him or her. "[The] patient is the ultimate judge of the value of the extra life which the treatment might provide."[3] While killing a dying patient may or may not be a compassionate act, allowing a dying patient to die is *always* compassionate. The treatments that clinicians may see as rescuing people, if only briefly, from imminent death may sometimes be experienced by patients and families as a torment from which they need to be freed.[4]

Eliminating the ethical and legal distinction between *killing* and *allowing to die* has profoundly dangerous implications. For instance, if the patient were dying from lack of treatment and not his or her fatal pathology, then withdrawing the treatment would be an instance of direct killing. We would be elevating the biological to an absolute value and we would be utterly ignoring the fundamental value of human life. We would be warehousing tens of thousands of people on ventilators and artificial nutrition and hydration. These people would be terribly vulnerable, unable to speak for themselves and trapped into involuntarily living by a spider's web of medical technology, permitted to die only after forty to sixty minutes of cardiopulmonary resuscitation is deemed to have failed. Death is not the worst thing. Involuntarily living is the worst thing.

For reasons of compassion as our rule, the only medical treatments that should *never be withheld or withdrawn* from a dying and suffering patient are the appropriate use of medications for symptom control and comfort care. With proper doses of comfort medications, the patient dies a *good death*–absent pain and suffering, both physical and existential–without being euthanized.

The moral intention in withholding or withdrawing life-sustaining treatment, allowing to die, is *not* the same as the moral intention in euthanasia. In euthanasia, we *intend* to kill the patient. In allowing a patient to die, we may say that "death is a blessing" or "let him be with God" or "let her die with dignity" but we do not intend the patient's death. We want the patient to live but only if his or her quality of life would be what she would want. We do not want the patient to suffer. We want our loved one back but only if she is healthy and whole.

Euthanasia–derived from the Greek *eu* (good) and *thanatos* (death), translating literally to *good death*–is, with no dissembling, a mercy killing. The term euthanasia in common usage now refers to a physician's action in accelerating a *good death* by the use of medications. Euthanasia happens, but so far, American society has not been willing to legalize it. In euthanasia, we intend to end the patient's suffering by ending the patient. We want the patient to be dead.

Often the terms *passive euthanasia* or *indirect euthanasia* are used to describe the withholding or withdrawing of life-sustaining treatment. Allowing a patient to die is not always morally wrong and is sometimes the only compassionate action. We must not confuse it with an action that seems morally wrong to most people. Therefore, we will not use the term passive euthanasia to refer to allowing a patient to die; we will reserve *euthanasia* for the active killing of a patient.

Although there may be a psychological difference between withholding and withdrawing life-sustaining treatment, there is no moral or legal difference. If it is *morally right* to withhold or forego a treatment in a certain set of circumstances, is it not morally right to withdraw that treatment in the same circumstances? A justification that is adequate for withholding a treatment is also sufficient for withdrawing it.[5] Otherwise, we would be forced to continue useless and unwanted treatment at the expense of the patient's well-being. If treatment that is started cannot be withdrawn, then we may well cause actual harm to a patient with absolutely no benefit.

Alternatively, if withholding and withdrawing are not morally equivalent, then there is a danger of under-treatment. This is an important point to consider, because when the prognosis is not clear, patients and surrogate decision-makers would rightly fear that treatment, once initiated, could never be withdrawn. The danger is that the patient or surrogate decision-maker would not allow life-sustaining treatment at all, and lives could be lost that otherwise might have been saved. If life-sustaining treatments could be withheld but not withdrawn, persons signing advance directives would refuse completely certain life-sustaining treatments, such as the use of a ventilator, when a ventilator might be life saving for a short period of a few days.[6]

A non-exhaustive list of examples of life-sustaining treatment that may be withheld or withdrawn are:

- Antibiotics
- Blood transfusions, blood products
- Cardiac catheterization
- Cardiopulmonary resuscitation
- Chemotherapy (unless palliative)

- Defibrillation devices

- Heart-lung bypass machines

- Hemodialysis

- Hydration (intravenous fluids)

- Mechanical ventilation, including ventilators and positive airway pressure devices (fixed-pressure CPAP and bi-level BPAP)

- Medications (i.e., vasopressors and anti-arrhythmics)

- Artificial nutrition delivered by tube (including total parenteral nutrition)

- Oxygen (except as for comfort)

- Pacemakers

- Radiation (unless palliative)

- Surgery (unless palliative)

- Organ transplants

Some less obvious example of life-sustaining treatment that may be withheld or withdrawn are:

- Placement (intensive care unit versus hospice)

- Central venous catheters for delivery of medications (portacaths, PICC lines, central lines)

- Diagnostic tests

- Monitors

Technology

If we are not going to try to cheat death, we do not need to know the results of diagnostic tests. If we are not going to treat whatever condition the diagnostic procedure is designed to detect, then we simply do not need to know about it. Many diagnostic tests can cause harm to fragile patients. An end-stage metastatic cancer patient in unrelieved pain cannot justifiably be transferred to a gurney to go to a scan. We do not need the information. All we need to know is that the patient is dying, and our only duty is to relieve pain and other symptoms.

Likewise, we do not need to watch monitors constantly. Often, when life-sustaining treatment is withdrawn in the intensive care unit, the family and friends gathered at the bedside watch the monitors for the flat-line and do not pay attention to their loved one. They miss the experience of accompanying their loved one to the end. They will come to regret it. A monitor may be on in the central station to aid healthcare providers in knowing when the patient dies.

In the intensive care unit, the patient generally has many diagnoses (some of which may be caused by other symptoms) and receives multiple life-sustaining treatments. In general, life-sustaining treatment is withdrawn in a certain sequence.

The general sequence of withdrawal is as follows:

- Hemodialysis
- Further diagnostic tests
- Vasopressors
- Intravenous fluids
- Hemodynamic and electrocardiographic monitoring
- Antibiotics
- Artificial nutrition
- Mechanical ventilation

Withholding antibiotics and dialysis is simpler because "the link between forgoing the intervention and death is not so obvious."[7] Withdrawing a ventilator is harder because the link to the patient not breathing and death is very obvious. Opioids such as morphine to reduce the subjective feeling of air hunger, and benzodiazepines or anti-anxiety agents, should be ordered in advance. The patient should be given a reasonable dose of these medications prior to the withdrawal of the ventilator to ensure comfort. Neuromuscular blocking agents, which paralyze the breathing muscles but do not alleviate air hunger, should never be used to make the patient "appear" comfortable for the sake of observers. After a ventilator is withdrawn and the patient survives for one to two hours, the patient should be transferred from the intensive care unit (ICU) to a medical-surgical unit for palliative treatment. ICU beds and ICU nurses are in short supply and those resources should be reserved for patients who will likely recover and walk out of the hospital. In addition, medical-surgical rooms generally are more comfortable for loved ones to gather.

Chapter 3. Ordinary and Extraordinary Treatment

Case 3-1 The Burn Patient.

Janny Jordan is a sixty-year-old woman with gall bladder cancer. She is a patient at a cancer hospital. Janny is offered an experimental chemotherapy by a physician who states that it "has a really good chance of curing your cancer or at least stopping it." Jenny considers her chance of cure and her quality of life after the treatment. She considers the side-effects and harms that the treatment could cause, which the physician describes as minimal nausea and vomiting. Janny accepts the risk. Janny receives one dose of the experimental chemotherapy and has a chemical burn that causes her epidermis to peel off. She acquires an infection and dies two days later.

Discussion Questions

- What could have motivated Janny's physician to recommend the experimental treatment that subsequently killed her?
- Might Janny's physician have had a personal motive for recommending the treatment?

In Chapter 1, we came to understand that a patient's quality of life is always determined by the patient. Quality of life is always specific and individual to the patient. This means that the determination of whether a treatment should be provided, withheld, or withdrawn, is also—and always—specific to the patient. The treatment *must* promote the quality of a patient's life. Different patients have different qualities of life and perceptions of how quality of life is understood. Even similarly situated patients, with all other things being equal, can have different qualities of life. We look toward a specific patient in a specific bed at a specific time and under a specific set of circumstances. A medical treatment must promote the quality of life of that specific patient. Therefore, while one medical treatment will benefit one patient's quality of life, the same treatment may frustrate another patient's quality of life. Because the provision of medical treatment is specific to the patient, we cannot *define* a standard by which to judge what treatment should be provided. However, we can *describe* the standard by which the patient and we can judge whether and what treatment should be provided—the basis is as contextual as it is individual.

When we discussed the difference between killing and allowing to die, we determined that our justification to provide, withhold, or withdraw life-sustaining treatment is always patient-centered. Just because a patient has lung cancer does not mean that she must undergo a second round of chemotherapy. However, another patient with the same cancer may choose to do so. It depends on the patient's evaluation of his own quality of life. If the patient evaluates that, with the treatment, he can live with an acceptable quality of life and can have a capacity to pursue his values, then the second round of chemotherapy may be appropriate. When the patient determines that the treatment will benefit his quality of life, we say that that treatment is *ordinary*. If the treatment will not benefit the patient's quality of life, we say that the treatment is *extraordinary*.

For centuries, bioethicists have been referring to the distinction between ordinary treatment, which is obligatory, and extraordinary treatment, which is optional. It is important to note that the terms *ordinary* and *extraordinary* are terms specific to clinical ethics, dating back to the 15th century, and, in this context, they do not have their ordinary meaning. Ordinary treatment is not the usual treatment or the customary treatment. Ordinary and extraordinary forms of treatment are not determined by classifying an intervention according to whether or not it is routinely used by reasonably prudent physicians. To the contrary, no intervention *in principle* is either ordinary or extraordinary because the treatment cannot be evaluated apart from the specific patient. Therefore, ordinary treatment is not normal hospital procedure. Ordinary treatment is not even the standard of medical practice. Just because we always do it does not mean that we should do it.

Sometimes bioethicists prefer *proportionate* or *disproportionate* to refer to ordinary and extraordinary treatment. However, these terms are somewhat misleading as there is no calculation; we do not know to what whole the proportion refers. Other bioethicists prefer *reasonable* or *unreasonable* treatment. However, these terms suggest that there is an objective, external criterion by which treatments will be judged obligatory or optional. There is no such thing. The terms *ordinary* and *extraordinary* are more accurate. The key to the distinction between ordinary and extraordinary treatments is *existential* because it refers to a patient's quality of life. It is not a purely *medical* distinction. Unfortunately, or fortunately, there is no *prima facie* definition of what are ordinary or extraordinary treatments.

The distinction between ordinary and extraordinary treatment is patient-specific. The historical, concrete, and specific characteristics of the patient and his quality of life are decisive. This is why there are no hard and fast rules to determine whether a treatment is ordinary or extraordinary. The determination is always made by the specific patient. A patient should never have to undergo treatment without consideration of the burdens that the treatment may cause, and a patient always may consider quality of life as opposed to prolongation of life solely for its own sake. As long as mere biological life is not the highest value, patients may consider the quality of their lives and choose to let their biological lives go.[1]

A patient determines whether a treatment is ordinary for him or herself. The patient considers his estimated quality of life after the treatment and the burdens that the treatment would impose. The patient determines what quality of life he is willing to live with, and the chances of achieving it, and whether the burdens of the treatment outweigh the benefits. Whether a treatment is ordinary or not is determined solely by the patient. A given patient may refuse a treatment that every other patient would choose to accept. If the patient chooses to refuse it, then it is extraordinary. For example, one patient may pursue extraordinary treatment in a research protocol. Another patient may forego the research protocol because the patient justly fears a profoundly diminished quality of life. What is at stake with the distinction between ordinary and extraordinary treatment is the patient's quality of life and the burdens of treatment, as perceived *by the patient*. Healthcare providers are profitably unjust to insist on extraordinary treatment that adversely affects the patient's perceived quality of life. To say otherwise is to deny the primacy of the patient.

Whether a treatment is ordinary or extraordinary is determined by those who have responsibility for the patient if the patient lacks the capacity to make the determination for him or herself. In this event, whether a medical intervention is ordinary is determined by its effect not only on the patient but also on those who have the responsibility to care for the patient. When a patient cannot care for him or herself, the emotional, physical, and financial burden to others needs to be included when assessing whether a treatment is ordinary or extraordinary.

When a patient, or those who have responsibility for a patient, determine that a treatment is not ordinary, but not futile, then the treatment is extraordinary. Extraordinary treatment either does not offer a reasonable hope of promoting a patient's perceived quality of life or imposes an unacceptable burden. To determine that a treatment is extraordinary, and need not be provided, is not to deny that the patient's life has value. When we forego extraordinary treatment, we are simply recognizing that either the proposed intervention does not promote the patient's quality of life or that the patient is dying. If the latter, then our only real obligation is to accompany the patient "to the gate," as it were. Mandating extraordinary interventions violates the patient's autonomy.

As we have seen, a treatment is either ordinary or extraordinary with regard to a specific patient. An abstract classification of technologies as ordinary or extraordinary apart from the patient is the wrong approach. For example, it is wrong to maintain that the key element in the traditional use of the distinction between ordinary and extraordinary treatment is the classification of the treatment—be it an application of technology, medication, or procedure. Further, it is wrong to categorize a treatment as ordinary solely because it is low technology and/or low risk, and it is wrong to classify a treatment as extraordinary because it is high technology and/or high risk. For example, artificial nutrition, once a gastrostomy tube is surgically placed in the abdomen, is low technology and carries low risk. A family member without any medical training can be taught to use the pump mechanism that delivers nutrients directly into the patient's stomach. However, artificial nutrition delivered by tube might be extraordinary and even harmful to an end-stage dementia patient.

Another example is a complicated surgical procedure on the heart requiring the use of a heart-lung bypass machine. The use of the heart-lung bypass machine may be ordinary for an otherwise healthy patient who will probably survive to see her young children grow up. The use of the machine may be extraordinary for a ninety-year-old woman who feels that she has lived a full and satisfactory life. The wrong contextual approach leads to the wrong conclusion. Once a treatment is classified according to the wrong approach, it may seem that the problem is resolved. However, we cannot consider the treatment apart from the specific patient. The distinction between ordinary and extraordinary treatments is determined by a process of *evaluation*, not as a classification of a treatment.[2]

There is an exception to the classification of treatment in principle. Comfort treatment for symptoms is always ordinary and never extraordinary. Symptoms to be aggressively treated include pain, dyspnea, nausea, vomiting, depression, anxiety, terminal agitation, and constipation (a common side effect of pain-relieving opiates). "Physicians should be skilled in the detection and management of terminal symptoms, such as pain, fatigue, and depression, and able to obtain the assistance of specialty colleagues when needed."[3]

Benefits and Effects

Medical effects are different from medical benefits. We treat whole patients: body, mind, heart, and spirit. We do not treat mere biological life and organ systems. The medical effect of a treatment is its impact on a patient's anatomy, physiology, chemistry, disease, organs, or pathological condition. The benefit of a treatment is understood as its effect on the whole patient and his ability to pursue their quality of life. The goal of medicine is to benefit the patient as a whole.

A patient must receive a net benefit for a medical treatment to be considered ordinary and morally obligatory. In other words, the benefit must be greater than the burden. Where benefit is represented by Be, and burden is represented by Bd: Be > Bd.

A treatment is considered beneficial if it:

- Restores health

- Reduces pain
- Restores consciousness
- Restores function
- Enables one to communicate with others
- Improves one's physical mobility
- Maintains life with reasonable hope of recovery
- Enables one to pursue life's purposes

A treatment is considered burdensome if it results in:

- Excessive suffering for the patient
- Financial hardship for the patient or the patient's family
- Emotional or physical burden to caregivers
- Excessive expense for the family, community, or society
- Inequitable allocation of a scarce resource, such as intensive care unit beds, according to principles of distributive justice
- An investment in medical technology and personnel disproportionate to the expected results
- No reasonable hope of benefit in promoting the patient's quality of life
- A profoundly frustrated quality of life

Note that the patient may actually be burdened by life-sustaining treatment. The patient may be suffering because of a decision to provide a medical effect for no benefit. Benefit and burden are relevant to quality of life, not to biological life.

Considering expense to the family and community is not the same as bedside rationing. Making decisions about life-sustaining treatment without consideration of the expense involved is unreasonable as long as we live in a world with limited resources. In the end, healthcare without cost effectiveness would become unaffordable to lower-income patients, offending distributive justice.[4]

We have no obligation to provide treatment that frustrates or eliminates the patient's quality of life when he cannot speak for himself. We have no obligation to treat a dying patient when medical treatment will only prolong the dying process. A patient's decision not to undergo extraordinary treatment is not morally equivalent to killing himself or herself. It reflects the patient's choice to recognize more important values than the value of mere biological life.

When a treatment cannot promote the patient's quality of life or would leave the patient in a condition where his quality of life is frustrated or eliminated altogether, then the treatment is considered extraordinary. In that case, the treatment offers only burden to the patient and is not in his best interests. The treatment has no positive goal. It may cause harm. The treatment has reached its limit and no longer fulfills its purpose. Comfort treatment must be provided and the patient must be allowed to die.[5]

Case 3-2. The Mistake.

Dr. Lu, an oncologist at a cancer hospital, meets with Harry and Elva Bean. Harry Bean is a seventy-five-year-old man with metastatic prostate cancer. Several chemotherapy agents have failed to stop the spread of his cancer, but Elva is unable to accept the fact that Harry is dying. After she cries in Dr. Lu's

office, Harry agrees to try again. Dr. Lu gives Harry a week's prescription to an oral chemotherapy agent. Harry returns to his home and takes the pills for three days. On the fourth day, Harry will not wake up when his wife shakes him. She calls 911. The paramedics find Harry to be unresponsive and unable to breathe. He is transported to the nearby community hospital where he is put on a ventilator. Harry dies two days later. His wife feels guilty that she pushed him to accept the aggressive treatment: "He was just fine until he had the pills. The doctor made a mistake. But it is my fault that he took the pills. I will never get over this."

Discussion Questions

- Did Harry's physician make a mistake in prescribing the oral chemotherapy?

- Why might Harry have taken the medication that he did not want? Do you believe that it is common for family members to persuade a patient to try to extend his life?

Case 3-3. The Burden to the Caregiver.

Morton is sixty-five years old. He has longstanding chronic kidney disease and blindness related to diabetes. He has received hemodialysis three times weekly for the last two years. He has been hospitalized five times since beginning hemodialysis for various issues, including: cardiac arrhythmias, hypotension, fluid overload, and pneumonia.

Morton is now bedbound and withdrawn. He lives at home with his son, George. Morton has expressed his wishes many times to not live in a skilled nursing facility, but his care at home has begun to be a heavy burden to his family. George has the financial stress of problems with his employer and is emotionally and physically exhausted. Neither George nor Morton has sufficient funds to hire a caregiver.

Morton has an advance directive that was executed fifteen years previously. It appoints his now-deceased wife, Jan, as his agent. The advance directive states that no life-sustaining treatment should be provided if he becomes permanently incapacitated.

George requests that the hemodialysis be withdrawn, and his father admitted to hospice so that he can have twenty-four hours a day access to skilled nurses and to the medications required to keep Morton comfortable during his dying process. Morton's physicians are uncomfortable with George's request, as they believe that his caregiver burden undercuts his decision-making. However, the ethics consultant points out that the healthcare team may consider the son's caregiver burden while supporting George's belief that continued life-sustaining treatment is extraordinary.

Discussion Questions

- Is Morton's hemodialysis extraordinary? Can it ethically be withdrawn?

- Does George have a right to consider the financial, emotional, and physical burdens that his father's continued life and care at home would demand of him?

- If George does not have a right to consider his caregiver burden, why not? What particular factors take precedence?

Chapter 4. Artificial Nutrition and Hydration

Case 4-1. The Tragedy of Terri Schiavo.

Theresa Marie Schindler Schiavo was born on December 3, 1963. On February 25, 1990, when she was only twenty-eight years old, she had a massive cardiac arrest at her home and was found by her husband, Michael. She was resuscitated but suffered immense anoxic brain damage from the lack of oxygen. She became comatose. After two and a half months without improvement, her diagnosis was changed to persistent vegetative state. She was cared for in a skilled nursing facility in Florida.

The persistent vegetative state is a mystery to most people. Persistent vegetative state patients are permanently unconscious and nonresponsive. However, their eyes are open and moving, they awaken and sleep, they move their facial muscles and smile and frown, and make sounds, sometimes appearing to laugh or cry. To the uninformed, and perhaps especially to the people who love them, persistent vegetative state patients appear responsive. However, they are not. Patients in the persistent vegetative state have no emotions, thoughts, ability to communicate, or self-awareness. They have no experiences. They do not sense the touch or presence of loved ones. They are permanently unaware of themselves or of their environments. No voluntary action, reaction, or behavior is present. Only the brain stem is alive, so reflexes and vegetative functions are present.

For two years, Michael took Terri to specialist after specialist, trying speech and physical therapies, including experimental therapies, in fruitless efforts to restore Terri to consciousness. In 1998, when Michael finally realized that Terri's condition would never improve, he petitioned the Sixth Circuit Court to have Terri's life-sustaining treatment withdrawn, namely the gastrostomy tube delivering artificial nutrition and hydration directly into her stomach. Michael, as Terri's legal guardian, believed that Terri would not want to live in a persistent vegetative state. Michael was opposed by Terri's parents, Robert and Mary Schindler, who believed that Terri's diagnosis was wrong and that she actively responded to them. They believed that Terri would not want her feeding tube to be withdrawn.

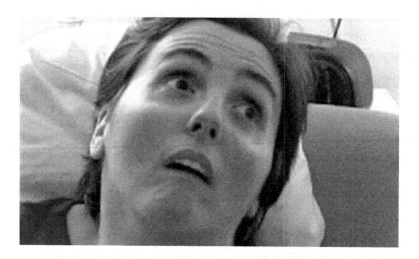

The Florida probate judge, Judge Greer, made two findings of fact. First, he ruled that Terri was in a persistent vegetative state and therefore unconscious and unaware. Second, he ruled that Terri would not want to prolong her life with artificial nutrition and hydration. He ordered the gastrostomy tube to be removed on April 24, 2001. It was withdrawn and then, due to the Schindlers' legal challenges, it was reinserted days later.

On February 25, 2005, Judge Greer again ordered removal of Terri's gastrostomy tube. The Schindlers appealed. They fought Michael through fourteen appeals and over one hundred motions, petitions, and hearings in the Florida courts. They fought with five suits in federal district court and four denials of certiorari from the United States Supreme Court, who refused to hear the case. Governor Jeb Bush signed an illegal law whose sole intent was to keep Terri alive. President George W. Bush returned to Washington D.C. to sign legislation designed to keep Terri alive. United States Congressmen, who did not understand the scientific complexity of the characteristics of a persistent vegetative state, argued that Terri was responsive.

The Schindlers also fought Michael for public sentiment. They took over two days' worth of video of Terri and selected a few minutes where she coincidentally appeared to respond. They placed the video on a website and argued that Terri was not in a persistent vegetative state. Disability rights, pro-life advocates, and religious figures were opposed by right-to-die advocates. Everyone held press conferences. The media reported that Terri was conscious and the removal of the gastrostomy tube was murder. Few articles in the media described disorders of consciousness. And yet, Michael persisted.

Finally, after the federal courts refused to interfere with the order to withdraw the artificial nutrition and hydration, the staff at Terri's hospice facility removed the gastrostomy tube on March 18, 2005. Terri died thirteen days later. An autopsy of her brain showed that it was half its normal size and there was such brain damage that she could not have been conscious. At no point did she respond to anyone or anything.

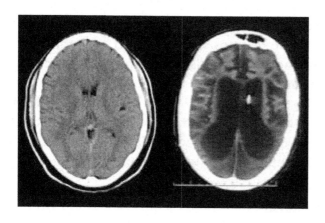

CT Scan image of Terri's brain (right) next to normal brain (left)

Jay Wolfson, the guardian ad litem appointed to represent Terri's interests, wrote emotionally about his involvement in Terri's case:

> During the thirty days of my report preparation, I spent about twenty with Theresa. I stayed with her for as long as four hours at a time, sometimes several times a day. I also spent time with her parents and siblings, with her husband, and with the governor, to whom I was reporting. My time with Theresa was emotional and intense. I sat with her, stood by her side, held her hand, stroked her hair, cradled her head in my hands, and looked deeply and closely into her eyes. I implored, cajoled, begged, and sought to find a consistent response, any response—anything other than reflex.[1]

Michael and the Schindlers fought over Terri's remains. Michael had Terri's body cremated and buried. Her headstone reads:

Schiavo / Theresa Marie / Beloved Wife

Born December 3, 1963

Departed this earth / February 25, 1990

At peace March 31, 2005

[Image of a dove with an olive branch]

I kept my promise

Conflicts between healthcare providers and a patient's surrogate decision-makers are especially likely with decision-making for patients who cannot swallow. These conflicts center on the use of artificial nutrition and hydration by nasogastric tubes, gastrostomy tubes, and intravenous lines. The primary examples of patients for whom artificial nutrition and hydration are at issue are patients in a persistent vegetative state and patients with end-stage dementia who are no longer able to swallow safely.

Patients in the Persistent Vegetative State

The persistent vegetative state is a mystery to most people. Persistent vegetative state patients are completely unaware of who and what is in their environment and do not respond to anything or anyone other than to painful and noxious stimuli. Persistent vegetative state patients do not experience hunger or thirst. They are permanently beyond experiencing physical suffering. The term *vegetative* is unfortunate, but it is the medically accepted term. We know that the persistent vegetative state patient is not a stalk of broccoli. We know that the biological lives of persistent vegetative state patients have the same fundamental moral value as our own.

The diagnosis of the lethal pathology, its persistence, means that the diagnosis of the persistent vegetative is also the prognosis. In this case, *persistent* means permanent. A persistent vegetative state patient will die of the persistent vegetative state. The fatal pathology prevents eating and drinking by mouth. A patient in a persistent vegetative state is in a condition that will lead to death regardless whether he or she receives artificial nutrition and hydration. Artificial nutrition and hydration merely prolongs the patient's biological life and hence the dying process.

A patient in the persistent vegetative state, receiving artificial nutrition and hydration and other medical treatments, is not physically suffering. However, the patient probably experiences existential suffering. He or she is living in the biological sense but has no quality of life. A persistent vegetative state patient is suffering by her very existence because he or she cannot pursue any purposes or values other than mere existence. Although the patient does not experience existential suffering *personally*, the patient's family and caregivers experience the transference tragedy so long as the patient's biological life continues with no quality of life present.

The persistent vegetative state is prolonged dying. The condition is a fatal pathology. The patient will die of her persistent vegetative state: the inability to swallow food and fluids, unless artificial nutrition and other life-sustaining treatments are given. If the patient is otherwise in good health and receives appropriate medical treatments, the patient can have a rather long biological life. Elaine Esposito lived in a persistent vegetative state for thirty-seven years. However, in the context of a persistent vegetative state, artificial nutrition and hydration will never promote a quality of life. Knowing what we know about quality of life, it must be true that most patients in the persistent vegetative state, were they able to miraculously regain decision-making capacity for the few minutes required to make a decision, would very likely not want their biological lives prolonged. As such, the provision of artificial nutrition and hydration is of no benefit and its withdrawal is of no harm.

Because artificial nutrition and hydration technology cannot restore a persistent vegetative state patient's quality of life, artificial nutrition and hydration are extraordinary treatments considering their lack of impact on a patient's quality of life. Those who advocate the withholding or the withdrawal of artificial nutrition and hydration from patients in the persistent vegetative state are not advocating killing. The intent is simply to end an extraordinary treatment. The patient experiences no benefit from artificial nutrition and hydration other than the preservation of her biological life. The intent in withholding or withdrawing artificial nutrition and hydration is to allow the patient to die. We release the patient from entrapment in her body. The patient in a persistent vegetative state is not capable of receiving any meaningful benefit from the efforts to preserve her biological life. The patient has no quality of life because the patient cannot pursue any human purposes whatsoever. Purely biological life can be let go.

Cardiopulmonary resuscitation, antibiotics, and artificial nutrition and hydration are extraordinary for the persistent vegetative state patient. These patients should be provided only supportive nursing care consistent with their human dignity. The decision to allow persistent vegetative state patients to die does not imply that their lives are less valuable than ours. The decision is because bare biological existence does not provide hope for any quality of life. There is no duty to preserve the biological lives of persistent vegetative state patients as they have no experiential quality of life to promote.

If artificial nutrition and hydration is withdrawn from a persistent vegetative state patient because it is extraordinary treatment, the patient's death is foreseen but the patient is not killed. The death occurs because artificial nutrition and hydration cannot correct the underlying fatal pathology: the permanent inability to ingest food and fluids orally. The death occurs because nothing gives the patient hope for any quality of life. Therefore, the withholding or withdrawal of artificial nutrition and hydration is not euthanasia.

Some people argue that artificial nutrition and hydration may never be withheld or withdrawn from a persistent vegetative state patient because it is *food and water*. However, they are confusing the *symbolic* meaning of food and water with a medical treatment that may be withheld or withdrawn just like any other medical treatment. The full meaning and associations of the term *food* are entirely human constructs. *Food* means the color, texture, aroma, taste, and indeed even the company in which it is shared. *Food* means shopping and cooking and eating. By contrast, a persistent vegetative state patient is fed involuntarily. Nutrition is administered to the patient's body and the patient's body absorbs it. The human symbolism of food is utterly absent.

Some argue that artificial nutrition and hydration is not a medical treatment subject to questions of ordinary or extraordinary treatment. They argue that artificial nutrition and hydration are basic elements of *care* and not medical treatments, and therefore, they must always be provided to a patient.[2] They argue that medical treatment aims at curing a clinically diagnosable condition but artificial nutrition and hydration are responses to "the basic needs of organisms to function and grow, not remedies of diseases in and of themselves."[3]

However, characterizing artificial nutrition and hydration as *care* does not automatically mean that it is obligatory. We need to define our understandings of *care*. The categorization of artificial nutrition and hydration as care is not an argument. As we explained in Chapter 3, no treatment can be categorized in principle as ordinary or extraordinary apart from the patient. Ordinary treatment and extraordinary treatment are determined only according to the specific patient's perspective and quality of life. Further, it is logically inconsistent to categorize nutrition and hydration as basic care because it is food and water and therefore a basic need, but then agree that mechanical ventilation is medical treatment. If food and water are basic needs, so is air, and it would be a tragic world indeed if we were never allowed to withdraw a ventilator.

People who adhere to the sanctity-of-life position and claim that biological life is the highest good, state that when we withdraw artificial nutrition and hydration from a patient in a persistent vegetative state, then we must intend to end that patient's alleged suffering by ending her life. They argue that this is euthanasia.[4] There is an alternative claim from the same position. Because a patient in the persistent vegetative state does *not* experience suffering because of artificial nutrition and hydration, the only intention we could have in discontinuing those medical treatments is to kill the patient by judging that he or she is undeserving of life. Yet we recall the distinction between killing and allowing to die. The intention is not to kill the patient but to stop providing medical treatment that has trapped the patient with no hope of escape and that violates that patient's human dignity.

Those who argue that the use of artificial nutrition and hydration is *care*, not medical treatment, state that the patient must always receive *care*. They state that whenever a medical device has been inserted or attached to a patient, and a layperson can be trained to use it, then the use of the device becomes nonmedical. When the device is nonmedical, it is in principle ordinary and must be used. With this logic, withholding a gastrostomy tube would be morally permissible as its insertion is a medical act. Withdrawing the device would be killing since the use of the device is not a medical act. However, we know that there is no ethical or legal distinction between withholding and withdrawing life-sustaining treatment. This means that there is also no ethical or legal distinction between withholding and withdrawing *care*.

The American Academy of Neurology states that while the placement of nutrients into a feeding tube is itself a relatively simple process and that the feeding does not require sophisticated mechanical equipment, that does not mean that the provision of artificial nutrition and hydration in this manner is a nursing rather than a medical procedure. The Academy points out that many forms of medical treatment, including, for example, chemotherapy or insulin treatments, involve the self-administration of prescription drugs by the patient. The Academy argues that these treatments are clearly medical, and their initiation and monitoring require medical attention. The position of the American Academy of Neurology is that once a patient has been reliably diagnosed as being in a persistent vegetative state and when the patient would not want further medical treatment, all further medical treatment, including the provision of artificial nutrition and hydration, may be withheld or withdrawn.[5]

A patient, or a person who speaks for a patient, may determine whether a treatment is ordinary or extraordinary depending on, amongst other factors: expense to the family, the community, and to society. Healthcare costs associated with artificial nutrition and hydration are significant. Terri Schiavo's medical treatment may have cost up to $100,000 a year and the cost of keeping all patients in persistent vegetative states in the United States may be as much as $9.25 billion per year. [6]

"The hidden issue in all of this is how much our society can afford to indulge this desire to keep people alive no matter what the cost."[7]

An article in *Neurology* on media coverage of the Schiavo case found that, of 1,141 relevant articles published between 1990 and 2005 in the four American newspapers with the highest circulation, twenty-one percent of the articles stated that Schiavo "might improve." Seven percent stated that she "might recover." Six percent explicitly denied Schiavo's persistent vegetative state diagnosis. Only one percent explained the persistent vegetative state or other chronic disorders of consciousness. In nine percent of articles, withdrawal of life support was described as murder. Most frequently cited descriptions of Schiavo's behaviors were: "Schiavo responds" (ten percent); "Schiavo reacts" (nine percent); "Schiavo smiles" (five percent); and "Schiavo laughs" (five percent). [8]

Yet polls show consistently that seventy to eighty percent of Americans would not want to be kept alive if they were in a persistent vegetative state or another irreversible coma-like situation. [9] Most Americans do not believe that these issues should be decided by politicians. In an ABC News poll taken while the Schiavo case was in the media, seventy percent of Americans said that it was inappropriate for Congress to get involved in the Schiavo matter, and sixty-seven percent thought that politicians were trying to keep Schiavo alive more for political gain than out of concern for her or a belief in the underlying principles. [10]

On the other hand, Not Dead Yet, a disability rights organization, objected to the withdrawal of artificial nutrition and hydration from Robert Wendland, a man in a minimally conscious state. [11] The court ruled that it was permissible to withdraw the artificial nutrition and hydration based on statements he had made while healthy. Not Dead Yet argued:

> Is pureeing food a medical treatment for a person who cannot eat solid food? Therefore, under the Appellate Court's ruling, could pureed food be withheld from an

elderly person who needs it to survive? When Medicaid pays for a personal assistant to help a person with quadriplegia eat, is that a medical treatment? Is giving liquid food through a tube in the mouth (a straw) a medical treatment? What if the tube is placed in the nose? In the throat? When does it stop being food and start being medicine? Can a surrogate similarly refuse a urinary catheter tube needed for waste elimination?[12]

Not Dead Yet's slippery slope argument does not consider whether feedings administered through a percutaneous gastrostomy tube, surgically placed in the stomach, is *food* or medical treatment.

Patients with End-Stage Dementia

Patients with end-stage dementia who survive to the point of being unable to swallow or who have lost all interest in eating and drinking are in the final phase of the disease process. This irreversible stage is the expected course of dementia. Many healthcare providers are convinced that artificial nutrition and hydration for dementia patients reduces wounds, reduces the risk of aspiration pneumonia, and prevents hunger and thirst. No data proves these claims. Research on artificial nutrition shows that it does not prevent aspiration pneumonia, skin breakdown, or wounds.[13] Furthermore, artificial nutrition can also result in increased and burdensome use of physical restraints to prevent dementia patients from pulling the tubes out of their abdomens, noses, or veins.[14] Artificial nutrition administered by vein or gastric tube may be withheld or withdrawn when the person with Alzheimer's disease or dementia is in the end stages of the disease and is no longer able to receive food or water by mouth. Of course, feeding by hand should always be attempted.

The benefits of artificial nutrition and hydration in end-stage dementia patients include eliminating the need for expensive hand feeding by medically trained staff and allowing reimbursement from Medicare, Medicaid, and private insurers. Potential risks of artificial nutrition and hydration, as indicated above, include restraints to prevent the patient pulling at the tubes, decreased human touch as hand feeding is eliminated, the continued risk of aspiration pneumonia from oral secretions and regurgitated feedings, and fluid overload.

The automatic reflex by a family and a physician to provide artificial nutrition and hydration for an end-stage dementia patient who cannot swallow is overwhelming. The common practice is to evaluate the patient's swallowing and if the patient can no longer swallow safely, to insert a nasogastric or gastrostomy feeding tube. Data shows that that placement of feeding tubes leads to the greater use of restraints, hospitalization for infections and aspiration pneumonia, and all without the prolongation of life.[15]

We need to recognize that the inability to take nutrition and hydration by mouth is usually an indication of the dying process for dementia patients.[16] Failure to recognize this process is to entangle patients in a nightmare of medical technology that they do not have the cognitive capacity to escape. Artificial nutrition and hydration is neither food nor water. It may be withheld or withdrawn like any other life-sustaining treatment. We need to stop the reflexive use of artificial nutrition and hydration in end-stage dementia patients that does not even prolong their biological lives. Most importantly, we need to stop tormenting them.

Terminally Ill Patients

Most terminally ill patients (for example, metastatic cancer patients) cease eating and drinking at the end. As the human body begins to die, the patient no longer experiences hunger or thirst. Lack of artificial nutrition and hydration is associated with decrease in tumor volume, with lessened end-stage congestion, less need for uncomfortable suctioning, and easier breathing. Finally, withdrawal or withholding artificial nutrition and hydration causes the body to release natural endorphins, natural morphine-like substances, allowing the patient to slip into a coma and die peacefully. Despite these benefits, families tend to feel guilt and anxiety if a patient is not eating or drinking, and hospice clinicians must educate them thoroughly and often about the patient's best interests.

Dehydration is how mammals die naturally. All mammals, including dogs, cats, and humans, who are allowed to die a natural death, stop eating and drinking. Ira Byock MD, director of Palliative medicine at Dartmouth Hitchcock Medical Center in New Hampshire, and author of the book, *Dying Well*, states: "The cessation of eating and drinking is the dominant way that mammals die. It is a very gentle way that nature has provided for animals to leave this life."[17]

Case Study 4-2 Expensive Nutrition for a Terminally Ill Patient.

Genevieve Logan is a thirty-three-year-old woman with metastatic breast cancer. Her primary care physician follows the generally accepted guidelines and does not order a routine mammogram for Genevieve. The cancer is found when Genevieve's partner notices a lump in her left breast.

Genevieve receives the standard treatment: mastectomy, with removal of the lymph nodes, chemotherapy, and radiation. However, after a week Genevieve refuses the cancer treatments because she is experiencing rashes, nausea, vomiting, and burns to her skin. Genevieve does not seek further treatment. Her oncologist loses touch with her after she begins to cancel appointments. Meanwhile, the cancer advances. Finally, Genevieve goes to the emergency room of the public hospital with abdominal pain and vomiting. She is found to have a bowel obstruction from metastasis.

A tube is used to pump gastric secretions from her intestine, preventing further vomiting and rupture of the intestine. However, because Genevieve's body cannot tolerate normal artificial feedings, the physicians order total parental nutrition (TPN). TPN is a liquid containing nutrition that is delivered directly into her bloodstream. The special nutrition solution used in TPN is very expensive. In addition, the provision of TPN by central venous catheterization is a relatively invasive procedure, which has risks of infection and septicemia.

Genevieve's physician recommends surgically circumventing the bowel obstruction and providing a gastrostomy tube. Artificial nutrition or even pureed food could be provided through the tube, eliminating the need for TPN. Genevieve agrees but the surgery ends when her surgeon observes tumors underlying the incision. Genevieve's entire abdomen is firm, indicating that it is full of tumors. It appears that there is not enough intact tissue for Genevieve to digest feedings. Thus, feeding by gastrostomy tube is impossible. TPN is continued. Meanwhile, Genevieve agrees to a Do-Not-Resuscitate (DNR) order. Cardiopulmonary Resuscitation (CPR) will not be provided if she suffers a cardiac arrest.

Genevieve's physicians begin to discuss withdrawing the TPN. One physician argues that the TPN should be withdrawn as it is expensive and is usually reserved for patients who have reasonable expectations of recovery. Genevieve has agreed to a DNR, because she herself has determined that CPR is an extraordinary treatment. This physician argues that because Genevieve does not want extraordinary treatment, she should not be treated with the TPN, even though there is no other way to provide her with nutrition. Another physician argues that TPN is food and not providing it would be tantamount to starving Genevieve painfully to death. However, the high cost of TPN is also an issue. Genevieve is in a public hospital and the taxpayers will ultimately pay any portion of her bill that Genevieve cannot pay.

Discussion Questions

- Is TPN, delivered through the bloodstream, food? Is withdrawing the TPN murder? Or is it withdrawing a life-sustaining treatment that is extraordinary?

- Is there a difference between pureed food delivered by a gastrostomy tube and TPN? What might the difference be?

- If the feeding tube had worked and Genevieve could have received pureed food directly into her stomach, would removing the feeding tube be withdrawing extraordinary treatment? Or would it be mercy killing?

- Cancer patients at the end of life frequently cannot assimilate nutrients however delivered. If Genevieve's body could not handle the TPN, it might just feed the tumors instead. Then would it then be appropriate to withdraw the TPN?

Chapter 5. Informed Choice

Case 5-1. The Appendix.

A nineteen-year-old woman named Suzette Martin goes to the emergency room of the local hospital. She is febrile and has severe pain that extends from her navel to the right side of her lower abdomen. She is also nauseous and vomiting. Suzette is diagnosed with acute appendicitis. Surgery is necessary. The surgeon visits Suzette and explains the procedure to be used. He describes what appendicitis is, the probable outcome of the surgery and the probable outcome with no surgery. He describes the surgery as immediately necessary if Suzette is going to live. Suzette asks if she can still have children after her appendix is removed.

Discussion Questions

- Suzette does not appear to understand the surgery that is recommended is an appendectomy and not a sterilization procedure. How might the physician explain?

- Does the fact that Suzette does not understand mean that Suzette should not make her own decision about the surgery?

If there can be said to be a single, universally shared human sentiment, it may well be this: that we all wish to die on our own terms. For this reason, patients must have the right to participate in decisions about their medical treatment. A specific patient makes the decision to use or forego a medical treatment based on the relationship between his medical condition and quality of life. The medical treatment must be consistent with the goal of medicine, to promote the patient's quality of life; preservation of mere biological life is not the true goal of medicine. The goal of medicine is to enable the patient to have a quality of life that is acceptable–and indeed, *appreciable*–to him or her. Therefore, a patient can refuse any or all life-sustaining treatments that only prolong his biological life. The patient has this right even when he will certainly die as a result of his choice.

Physicians use their knowledge, experience, and training to determine the patient's diagnosis. However, determining root specificity for the diagnosis is not always possible save by an autopsy. For example, the physician may diagnose a cancer metastasis but not know where the primary cancer is located. No diagnostic test should be performed if the patient is irrevocably dying and beyond hopeful treatment options. For the purposes of the goal of medicine, we really do not need to know any more than the fact that the patient is dying of the metastasis. Conversely, a patient may have five or even ten diagnoses at the same time.

Physicians also use their knowledge, experience, and training to determine the patient's prognosis–including both the estimated *quantity* of life and the probable *quality* of that life. Determining prognosis may often be far simpler than determining diagnosis.

Commonly, we often say that the patient consents to or refuses a specific treatment. This is generally called *informed consent*. However, we use the term *informed choice* to reflect that an informed patient may consent to or refuse a treatment. Informed consent reflects only one choice of treatment. The physician should offer more than one option. The options must include at least one treatment that the patient may choose, as well as the option of no treatment. Therefore, the patient chooses among at least two options. He does not consent to only one course of action.

Once, decisions about treatment were made by physicians alone. The decision-making rationale was opaque to the patient. This model of decision-making is a paternalistic model.[1] The physician acted as the father and the patient was treated as the child. The patient did not contribute toward the decision. There was always potential for abuse under the paternalistic model.

The informed consent model of decision-making limits the role of the physician to giving the patient information. The patient has the ultimate control. This is called the *patient consumer* model. The patient makes an autonomous choice and is responsible for the consequences of that choice.

The shared decision-making model acknowledges the power differential that exists between the physician and the patient. The patient is vulnerable and depends on the physician. The physician may hold life or death in her hands.

The shared decision-making model depends on the involvement of both the patient and the physician. This means that the patient must be able not only to choose a treatment, but that this choice is informed. The shared decision-making model also acknowledges that the flow of information is asymmetrical. The physician knows the medical science. The patient knows his values. Only the physician knows how the treatment option in question acts on the patient's medical condition. The patient, on the other hand, knows how his medical condition affects his quality of life. For the patient to make a truly informed choice to choose or to refuse a medical treatment requires both kinds of information. Therefore, the shared decision-making acknowledges both the power differential and the asymmetric information between the physician and the patient.

The physician informs the patient about the risks and benefits of each option, *always* including the option of no treatment. The patient then determines what risks and benefits he is willing to accept. The physician must take care to explain the medical information and makes certain that the patient understands his assumptions about the information. The physician must transfer information along with a way of thinking about the information so that the patient can make an informed choice (more on this vital aspect later).

In the shared decision-making model, the physician also elicits the patient's values. The physician and the patient then use the patient's own values to discern which treatment, or no treatment, best promotes the patient's quality of life. Examples of the patient's values may include: improved function, elimination of pain, short recovery time, and so on. The physician may believe that the patient would be better off with a treatment that the patient does not choose. However, the physician must present the treatment options in-line with the patient's values, not the physician's.

We must understand—a recommendation by a physician is *extremely* powerful. With a recommendation, the physician directs the patient how to think through the available information, especially including treatments with uncertain benefits and risks. "The physician has an ethical obligation to help the patient make choices from among the therapeutic alternatives consistent with good medical practice."[2] The physician cannot lay out a smorgasbord of alternative treatments, including their myriad risks and benefits, and expect the patient to make an informed decision without a recommendation of the best course forward. The physician must *help* the patient make an informed decision.

A recommendation should answer the following questions:

"What would you do if you were me?"

"What if she were your grandmother?"

"What decision would you make for yourself?"

Informed choice is a process of communication, far more than just a patient's signature on a hospital consent form. The vital communication between a physician and a patient's results in the patient's consent or refusal to accept a specific medical treatment. A hospital consent form is not *itself* informed consent. It is just a piece of paper. A patient's signature on a form does not mean that there was really consent or that it was informed. Legally, the signed consent form is only *presumed* valid. Later evidence may show that the consent was not informed, as is often the case with challenged consent documents.

The patient has an informed choice to consent to, or refuse, a medical treatment. In order to choose, the patient requires appropriate and consistent information, preferably including all of the below:

- The patient's diagnosis, if known.
- The patient's prognosis, including the patient's probable future medical condition.
- The nature and purpose of the proposed treatment.
- The risks, benefits, and uncertainties of the proposed treatment.
- Reasonable alternatives to the proposed treatment or procedure including the patient's probable medical condition after undergoing each alternative treatment.

- The risks and benefits of not receiving or undergoing the treatment.

- A recommendation by the treating physician regarding the treatment, including sharing her reasoning process with the patient, and informed by the patient's quality of life.

- The assessment of patient understanding and capacity to make a decision.

- The consent or refusal of the treatment by the patient.

Note that we strive to *never* inform a patient about treatments that will be futile and that therefore cannot be performed. We never ask if the patient wants "everything done" as ethically, "everything done" means everything *reasonable*, not everything *possible.* Admittedly, to a patient or a patient's loved ones, "everything" may well mean something quite different.

In many medical situations, a patient may receive inconsistent information from many different sources, including his attending physician, consultant specialists, primary care provider, and interns and residents if applicable. Some physicians are more consistent than others in providing information or are more able to communicate in a way that the patient can understand. Other physicians unfortunately use medical jargon without explanation or substitute laboratory findings for pertinent information. Some clinicians lay out a whole set of alternative treatments without actually making a recommendation and somehow expect the patient to make a rapid decision. For most patients under these circumstances, making an informed decision is simply impossible. To perform ethically, the physician recommending a particular treatment or procedure must ensure that the patient is adequately informed, adequately understands, and chooses freely.

There are three standards to determine if *informed choice* is met:

- The reasonable physician standard
- The reasonable patient standard
- The subjective standard

The reasonable physician standard is what a typical physician would disclose about the proposed treatment. However, a typical physician may not give a specific patient all the information required to make an informed decision. The reasonable physician standard does not guarantee an informed choice. The focus here is inappropriately on the *physician* knows, rather than on what the *patient* needs to know.

The reasonable patient standard involves what the typical patient would need to know in order to make an informed decision. The issue here is that it ignores the specific needs and conditions of the patient. This is why cultural and language interpreters are so important. Our explanation may be designed to be understood by a white, middle-class, English-speaking patient with a college degree. Our explanation may be utter gibberish to a patient who only speaks his native language and is of a culture that we may not understand or who has a low level of health literacy. In such cases, the reasonable patient standard is not just and it is not kind.

In addition, relying on a family member to translate for a non-English speaking patient puts undue pressure on the family member translating. It also allows the family member to "protect" the patient by withholding information. Some people come from cultures where a cancer diagnosis is traditionally hidden from a patient. Other patients come from cultures in which the patriarch of the family or the eldest son makes the decisions. In these cases it is helpful, through a translator, to ask the patient what information she wants and who she wants to make the decision. Some cultures and religious traditions are more likely to forego decision-making in favor of the physician's recommendation.

The subjective standard asks what *this specific patient* would need to know and understand in order to make an informed decision. This standard is the most challenging to use because it requires tailoring information to each patient. However, it is the only standard that guarantees that the patient can make an informed decision. A patient making a decision about treatment needs the information presented in a way the patient can understand. "The quantity and specificity of this information should be tailored to meet the preferences and needs of individual patients."[3] Note that many institutional risk managers hate the subjective standard as it is necessarily *ad hoc*.

Under the subjective standard, the patient must fully understand the information provided before he can make an informed choice. Consequently, the discussion should be carried on in layperson's terms and the patient's understanding of each component of the information should be separately assessed. Often the physician just needs patience, repeating the necessary information and allowing time for the patient to absorb things, or allowing the patient to discuss the information with others. Patient understanding may require eliminating medical jargon, including laboratory values. It may require a diverse approach - communicating orally, in video, in writing, as well as presenting information at the appropriate reading level. Extra time and resources must be used with patients who have low health literacy. We must use interpreters who have special expertise in the patient's culture and language. Some hospitals have interpreters on staff while others may use translators on dual headset telephones.

We must be also careful about a patient who nods his head affirmatively when the physician speaks and yet asks no questions when invited to do so. It is one thing to rely on a physician's recommendation but another entirely to agree blindly with everything the physician says. Only in emergency situations should the patient's choice should be presumed rather than obtained—when the patient is unconscious or incapacitated and no surrogate decision-maker is available.

There are more malpractice cases over lack of informed choice than over actual medical errors. If a physician notifies a patient of the possible risks and harms of the proposed treatment and those risks and harms materialize then, assuming there were no medical errors, there has been no medical malpractice. If the physician fails to inform the patient of the possible risks and harms and they materialize, then the physician has committed malpractice—not due to any specific error but because of failure to provide the patient with the chance to make an informed choice. An outcome should never surprise a patient.

Case 5-2. Nodding Yes.

An elderly man named Wei Zhao visits a local clinic. The admitting nurse takes his blood pressure. It is very high. She tells the physician immediately. The physician speaks to Wei Zhao about the danger of high blood pressure and the risk of not treating it. He also describes the benefits and risks of different treatments. Wei Zhao nods his head yes and smiles during the physician's explanation. Wei Zhao leaves with a prescription. The office manager realizes that Wei Zhao speaks no English when she cannot make him understand that he needs a follow-up appointment.

Discussion Questions

- Has Wei Zhao made an informed choice to accept treatment for his hypertension?

- How might the physician make certain that Wei Zhao understands his condition and the proposed treatment?

Chapter 6. Decision-Making Capacity

Case 6-1. Afraid of the Doctor.

Maryann Barry is an eighty-six-year-old widow who lives in an assisted living retirement home in California. She has no living family, but she does have one good friend who lives nearby. Maryann is in the hospital for treatment of a urinary tract infection from which she is recovering. However, she also has renal disease and has been on hemodialysis for two years.

For at least the past eight months, Maryann has told her dialysis nurses and her friends at the retirement home that she wants to stop the dialysis. However, she faithfully goes to the dialysis center three times each week. Maryann claims that her nephrologist refuses to listen when she tells him that she wants to stop dialysis.

Maryann is admitted to the hospital with heavy diarrhea. She continues to say that she wants to stop dialysis. However, when Maryann's nephrologist visits her in the hospital she is quiet and appears to accept treatment. With others, she complains urgently and tearfully that she wants to stop dialysis.

Discussion Questions
- Does Maryann have the ability to make the decision to stop dialysis?
- If so, why can't she make a decision?
- What factors are influencing her ability to make a decision?

Several factors influence a treating physician's determination as to whether the patient has the capacity to decide to consent to or refuse a particular treatment. These factors include: assessing the patient's capability, the requirements for making the decision, and how the decision will affect the patient's medical condition. In the end, however, the patient decides whether the treatment promotes or frustrates his quality of life.

If a patient has decision-making capacity, then he can determine if a specific treatment is ordinary or extraordinary. Respect for the dignity of the patient requires that, where at all possible, the patient be empowered to make his own decisions. The exceptions are decisions for which he lacks specific capacity. A patient is always presumed to have decision-making capacity unless evidence shows otherwise.[1]

We have to be absolutely clear that decision-making capacity is *not* the same thing as competence. *Capacity* is a clinical term that is specific to a particular decision. *Incompetency* is a legal determination by a probate judge that a person lacks the ability to make all of his or her own decisions.

The concept of capacity is precise and patient-centered. The capacity that we measure is the ability of the specific patient to make a specific decision. Capacity is always relative to a decision, always specific to a task. Therefore, *capacity* always refers to *the capacity to* make a particular decision. Capacity requirements vary considerably according to the decision.[2]

The level of capacity required to make a specific decision varies according to several factors. There is variation in the decision's objective as well as in the patient's ability to meet those demands.

- A patient may be able to make one type of decision and not another.

- A patient may be able to make a decision at one time and not another.

- A patient may be able to make a decision under one set of conditions and not another.

- A patient may be able to make a decision depending on the latest dose of medication.

- A patient may be able to make a decision during one hospital admission but not a subsequent admission.

- A patient may be able to make a decision depending on who is asking the question.

- A patient may be able to make a decision in one environment and not another.

- A patient may be unable to make a decision for a myriad of medical issues, including deprivation of oxygen, metabolic disturbances, and infection.

Degrees of capacity can vary widely according to the patient's nature in the intimidating, unfamiliar, and stressful hospital environment or even according to who is asking the question. The patient's trust in the physician should be assessed honestly. A patient receiving hemodialysis, for example, may tell her friends and her nurses repeatedly and emotionally that she wants to refuse dialysis, but may be sufficiently intimidated by her nephrologist to continue to go to the dialysis center three times a week. In this case, the patient lacks capacity to make a decision about proceeding with dialysis or refusing it because she fears the physician ordering it.

The patient must have the capabilities required for making the specific decision:

- The patient must be able to understand both the potential risks of harm and benefits of alternative interventions.

- The patient must be able to communicate the decision.

- The patient must be able to communicate his reasons for the decision.

- The patient must be able to imagine what it would be like to undergo various experiences related to treatment.

- The patient must be able to draw inferences about the consequences of making a given choice.

- The patient must be able to compare alternative outcomes based on how they promote or frustrate the patient's quality of life.

In order to meet the demand of a decision, the patient must have a set of values that is at least "minimally consistent, stable, and affirmed as his own."[3] The patient must have a stable set of values in order to evaluate particular outcomes as they affect his quality of life. The patient must also be able to allocate relative importance or weight to these outcomes. Ultimately, the patient must be able to match his values to particular treatment alternatives in order to determine what treatments are ordinary or extraordinary for himself.

The question of capacity is a straight-forward, yes or no determination.[4] Capacity is an all-or-nothing concept, not a comparative concept. The function of capacity determinations is to sort people into two very distinct groups. One group consists of those patients who demonstratively *have the capacity* to make a particular decision that we, as medical professionals, have a duty to respect. The other group is patients *who lack the capacity* to make a particular decision, where the decision will be made by others. Capacity is both decision and individual-specific. The patient's capacity *must* be considered as foremost with regard to every decision.

Setting the proper standard of decision-making capacity involves two values: the patient's self-determination and the patient's well-being. In balancing these two values, it is important to avoid failing to protect the well-being of an incapacitated patient or fail to respect the self-determination of a patient with capacity. The looser the standard for capacity, the more common it is to fail to protect the patient's well-being; the stricter the standard of capacity, the more common it is to fail to respect the patient's self-determination.[5] Deciding how to set the standard for capacity so that it avoids both types of errors is not a factual matter. It is a reasonable choice of values.[6]

There are three standards for informed choice and–as we've covered–two standards of capacity. In regards to the former, the first is the outcome standard. To meet this standard, the decision must be one that a "reasonable" patient would make. The decision must be compared to a decision by a similarly situated, fully cognizant patient. The patient's decision is evaluated according to an objective and external standard. A decision that does not meet this standard is evaluated as an incapacitated choice. However, the outcome standard ignores the specific patient's quality of life, which presents an issue. "Any standard of individual well-being that does not ultimately rest on an individual's own underlying and enduring aims and values is both problematic in theory and subject to intolerable abuse in practice."[7] As all attorneys know, it is notoriously difficult to determine who the reasonable person is. Is it you, or your mother-in-law, or your high school basketball coach?

The second standard of capacity is the process standard. The process standard involves assessing the process that the patient uses to arrive at a decision. It does not assess whether the decision the patient makes is the one recommended by the physician. It also does not test the patient's decision against that of a "reasonable" patient. The process standard involves answering the following two questions:

> "How well must the patient understand and reason to have capacity?"

> "How certain must the persons be who are testing that capacity?"[8]

Whether the process standard is met depends in large part on the treatment's potential benefits and its risk of potential harms. A risk-benefit determination should always be made with regard to a treatment in order to determine if a patient has the decision-making capacity to choose it or to refuse it. "Risk is the product of the magnitude of the harm that would result from the decision and the probability that the harm will result if the decision is followed."[9] The physician offering the treatment is responsible for determining potential benefit and risk of harm if the patient chooses or refuses the treatment.

Different decisions with different potential benefits and potential harms require different levels of decision-making capacity. Under the process standard, the level of capacity required to make a particular decision about treatment ranges from low to high depending on the potential benefits and risks of harms of the treatment. The more serious the expected risk to the patient from acting on a choice, the higher the standard of capacity should be; as well, the certainty of assurance that the standard is satisfied must rise. For example, the patient needs more capacity to make a life-and-death decision than he may for less drastic decisions. This also means that a patient may have capacity to consent to a treatment but lack capacity to refuse it.[10]

If the potential benefits and harms analysis is favorable and the patient consents to the treatment, then a relatively low level of capacity is required. Likewise, if the risk-benefit is unfavorable and the patient refuses, a low level of capacity is sufficient to sustain the decision. If the risk-benefit analysis is intermediate and balanced, regardless of whether the patient consents or refuses, an intermediate level of capacity is required. If the risk-benefit analysis is favorable and patient refuses, or if the risk-benefit analysis is unfavorable and patient consents, then a high level of capacity is demanded, as well as a high certainty that the standard is met.[11]

For example, a "pleasantly confused" patient with dementia might be able to decide that she wants a certain type of medication that might make her sleepy and prevent her from spending time with her family, assuming that its burdens and risks are low. However, the same patient might be unable to weigh the risks and benefits of a cardiac surgery with alternative outcomes which would profoundly affect her values of quantity and quality of life. Likewise, an otherwise healthy patient—without religious or cultural prohibitions affecting the decision—would need a high level of capacity for refusing a life-saving surgery with few risks, but a low level of capacity to consent to it. Note that a patient may lack capacity to make a decision about surgery but still may have capacity for lesser decisions, such as designating a surrogate decision-maker.

Consider an eighty-year-old patient with dementia who develops life-threatening pneumonia. If she is still awake and aware, albeit demented, she may have the capacity to agree to ventilator treatment to save her life, but lack the capacity to refuse it and allow herself to die. This does not mean, however, that she should necessarily receive ventilator treatment. The patient's family and friends may indicate that the patient is an independent-minded person who would never want ventilator treatment if she had to die with it.

Sometimes a refusal of treatment may reasonably trigger capacity investigation, but only when the patient is unwilling to discuss her reason for the refusal of treatment, or the refusal is based on "misunderstanding or irrational biases."[12] However, the refusal of treatment itself is not alone conclusive evidence that the patient lacks capacity. According to the process standard, we need to evaluate the *process* by which the patient came to the decision, not just the outcome. A patient's rejection of a physician's recommendation should not trigger an evaluation of the patient's capacity if the patient chooses another treatment that equally or better promotes his quality of life.

Decision-making capacity should be investigated under two conditions. First, capacity should be determined when a patient makes the recommended choice but the outcome adversely affects the patient's quality of life; second, a capacity investigation should be triggered when the patient agrees to a treatment blindly, without sufficiently understanding the risks and benefits, the alternatives, and the consequences of that decision. In that case, the patient may have capacity but may have simply decided to follow the physician's recommendation.[13]

In an investigation into a patient's decision-making capacity, the physician must ask several questions:

- What does the patient understand about his medical condition?

- What is the patient's understanding of how his medical condition relates to his quality of life?

- What is the patient's level of understanding about the risks of harm and the benefits from the recommended treatment and alternative treatments?
- Why does the patient believe that the physician has recommended the treatment?
- What does the patient think will actually happen if the patient consents to the treatment or refuses it?

Marc Tunzi suggests some very good questions to help evaluate patient capacity, including:

"Why do you think your doctor has recommended [proposed] treatment?"

"Do you trust your doctor?"

"What do you think will happen to you now?"[14]

Not only should the patient have the capacity to make the decision in question, the patient also needs to stick to that decision. If a patient cannot make up his mind and his decision about the treatment vacillates wildly, then the patient demonstrates a lack of decision-making capacity.

While decision-making capacity and cognitive ability are correlated, they are not the same thing. Cognitive impairment does not necessarily equal a lack of decision-making capacity. Decision-making capacity refers to the patient's ability to make a particular decision. Cognitive ability encompasses the entirety of the patient's attention span, memory, and problem-solving abilities. A patient may have diminished cognitive ability but still have capacity to make low-risk, low-harm decisions—such as whether to agree to antibiotics for a urinary tract infection.

One important point to make at this juncture is that tests of cognition do not substitute for a specific capacity assessment. False results from cognitive tests such as the Mini Mental State Examination (MMSE) are quite common. The MMSE frequently shows false positives for vulnerable and disadvantaged patients. It also tends to produce false negatives for highly educated patients with highly developed reasoning skills.[15] Failure of a cognitive test should only trigger more assessment, *not* decide the question. In addition, the input of psychiatrists and psychologists is not always necessary to determine capacity.[16] The responsibility lies with the physician proposing the treatment. Nurses, clinical social workers, and chaplains may be able to provide facts and insights that aid the physician in determining the patient's capacity.

A patient who has capacity has the fundamental right to make an irrational decision. A surrogate decision-maker does not. For our purposes, an *irrational decision* is a decision that satisfies the patient's own values less completely than other available choices. A patient with capacity who wishes to go on living a healthy, productive life yet refuses a low-risk, low-harm, life-sustaining intervention has made an irrational choice. Yet, if the patient is determined to have capacity, we must respect the patient's choice, regardless if the decision appears by all measures an irrational one. Again, we must accept that a patient with capacity has the right to make an irrational decision. Moreover, a patient's decision may appear irrational at first glance but, after a detailed discussion, may be merely unusual or idiosyncratic—not genuinely irrational. A patient may refuse to undergo a colonoscopy even if it will prevent a much worse experience, such as cancer treatment or even death, for reasons that are entirely his own. A capacity determination can be triggered *only* if the patient refuses to discuss his reasoning for the refusal.

To paint an example: an adult patient who is a Jehovah's Witness may refuse blood products even at the cost of his life. The refusal may seem utterly irrational to us, while it is perfectly rational to the patient. If blood products are administered, the patient will forfeit his salvation. Conversely, the young child of Jehovah's Witness parents does not have the decision-making capacity to refuse a life-saving and low-risk blood transfusion.

Magical thinking is the belief that an object, action, or circumstance that is not logically related to a course of events can influence its outcome. Decisions due to magical thinking are a major category of irrational decisions. Magical beliefs can affect decision-making in some of the following ways:

- A patient with a family history of colon cancer refuses a colonoscopy because he fears that it will uncover colon cancer: "If I don't know I have it, I don't have it."

- A patient refuses a colonoscopy because colon cancer "won't happen to me."

- A patient refuses a colonoscopy from an unreasonable fear that "being put to sleep" or "being cut open" will result in death. (However, the realistic risk of death is part of the information needed for informed consent.)

- A family insists on futile treatment for their loved one because they are "waiting for a miracle."

If the patient makes choices that just do not make sense, we respect the decision if it accords with a well-recognized—though perhaps unusual—belief or cultural value. However, when the decision is not attributable to a recognizable religious belief or cultural value, we respect the decision if it is, nevertheless, a strongly held value. In this case, we must determine if the seemingly irrational decision is due to a distortion of values caused by a treatable condition, such as depression.

On the other hand, a surrogate decision-maker may not make an irrational decision. It is irrational to refuse to allow the withdrawal of a ventilator for a ninety-year-old patient who is in failing health, has sepsis, and end-stage dementia, because the treatment is only prolonging the patient's inevitable death and is causing active suffering. It is irrational to insist on artificial nutrition for a dying loved one because "God has to have time to work a miracle." A *patient* with decision-making capacity may irrationally demand life-sustaining treatment in the hopes that God will work a miracle. A surrogate *may not* torture a patient because the surrogate is waiting for a miraculous healing.

Case 6-2. They are Trying to Kill Me!

Jermaine Hopkins is sixty years old. He has bipolar disorder that is being treated with medication. Due to a complication of diabetes, Jermaine has received hemodialysis three times a week for a year. His renal failure is not improving, and he realizes that he will be on dialysis three times a week for the rest of his life. After considerable anguish, Jermaine decides to discontinue dialysis. Dialysis is extraordinary for Jermaine and frustrates his quality of life. He resents having to go to the dialysis center three times a week for six hours at a time. Jermaine cannot do anything that promotes his quality of life on the four days that he is not at the center because he is too tired. Jermaine requests discontinuing the dialysis and going to the palliative care unit of his local hospital for comfort care.

Within three days of discontinuing dialysis, Jermaine becomes agitated and delirious and believes that his healthcare team is trying to murder him. Confused, Jermaine states that he wants to resume hemodialysis. The attending physician and other members of the healthcare team determine that Jermaine now lacks capacity to make the decision to resume hemodialysis and should remain in palliative care with comfort measures only. The ethics consultant speaks with Jermaine. Jermaine's speech is rapid and pressured, and he appears to be extremely anxious, perhaps triggered by his renal failure. He manages to calm down somewhat when the palliative care nurse practitioner convinces him that no one is going to kill him.

The ethics consultant points out that the decision to resume life-sustaining treatment requires less capacity than to refuse it. The ethics consultant recommends that hemodialysis be resumed, and a further conversation be had with Jermaine about withdrawing it again. This conversation should include what Jermaine wants to happen if he again becomes delirious.

Discussion Questions

- Does Jermaine's anxiety influence his capacity to make a decision about stopping dialysis?
- Did Jermaine lose his capacity to make a decision over the period of time between his initial refusal of dialysis and the time when the ethics consultant speaks to him?
- If so, why should we start dialysis again?

Case 6-3. What Do You Want?

Jennifer White is a sixty-seven-year-old woman with metastatic colon cancer. She goes to the emergency room of her community hospital with severe abdominal pain and vomiting. In the emergency room, Jennifer states that her husband, Thomas, should make all decisions if she becomes incapacitated. She tells her admitting physician that she has no advance directive and she does not want one. She states that she trusts her husband to make the right decisions for her. She also states that she wants all life-sustaining treatment, including cardiopulmonary resuscitation (CPR). She is admitted to the hospital for treatment of a small bowel obstruction.

During her hospitalization, Jennifer's cancer advances and her medical condition deteriorates rapidly. She now requires several life-sustaining treatments, including a positive airway pressure device and high doses of intravenous vasopressor medications to maintain her blood pressure.

Jennifer's attending physician reviews her treatments and her medical condition with Jennifer. He tells Jennifer that she has a "poor prognosis for survival." Jennifer pins her physician down and he finally admits that Jennifer is dying. Jennifer's response is to continue all of her current life-sustaining treatments. She also wants full aggressive treatment in case there is another, future problem. Jennifer repeatedly says: "I don't want to let my family down." Her physician supports her but does point out that Jennifer is at a high risk of not being able to breathe and that her heart is rapidly failing. The physician states that CPR would not only be ineffective, it would cause her to suffer as she dies.

Jennifer agrees that she does not want CPR yet she refuses to sign a Do-Not-Resuscitate (DNR) order. Her physician asks her again a few days later. Jennifer repeats that she does not want to be resuscitated but again refuses to sign the DNR. The physician holds a family conference in Jennifer's room, including Thomas and the couple's two adult children. When her physician asks Jennifer to discuss with her family why she does not want CPR, Jennifer denies that she ever said such a thing.

The next day, Jennifer admits to her physician that she lied in order to spare her family the pain of knowing that *she* knows that she is dying. Jennifer's physician speaks to Thomas privately. Thomas states that he wants CPR even though he knows that it would make Jennifer suffer. He wants to prolong her life as long as possible, even for a few minutes, and under any circumstances. A day later, Jennifer stops breathing and her heart stops.

Discussion Questions

- How do we interpret Jennifer's ambivalence about CPR?
- Under the circumstances, did Jennifer have the capacity to make a decision about CPR?
- Now that her heart is stopped, do we attempt to resuscitate Jennifer or not?
- Would an attempt to resuscitate Jennifer work?

Chapter 7. Decision-Making for Incapacitated Patients

Case 7-1. Who Makes the Decision?

A middle-aged, alcoholic, homeless man falls to the pavement on Skid Row with what is later diagnosed as a hemorrhagic stroke. The patient is transported to the public hospital and receives ventilator treatment and artificial feedings. He is unresponsive. He has no gag reflex and does not react when the neurologist pinches him. The hospital social worker asks the police to fingerprint the homeless man. When the prints come back, the man is identified by his criminal record as Gerald Smith. The social worker searches the available databases and finds one family member: David, Gerald's son.

David is furiously estranged from Gerald. Gerald was "a falling down, dead drunk" when David was a child and he physically, emotionally, and verbally abused both David and his mother. David's co-dependent mother always made excuses for Gerald's abusive behavior, which further angered David. David left the home when he was fourteen and moved in with his maternal grandmother. She died two years later and David was on his own from then on.

David is of two minds when asked if he will make the decision to remove Gerald from the ventilator and allow him to die. On one hand, David hopes that Gerald is suffering and believes that he should remain on the ventilator so that he can continue suffering. On the other hand, David wants an apology. After years of therapy, David knows rationally that he will never hear an apology from Gerald. Yet he cannot quite let Gerald die without getting one. David's first emotional inclination is to demand that Gerald's life be prolonged as long as possible.

However, after much discussion with his priest and his therapist, David takes himself into hand and permits Gerald's ventilator to be withdrawn. Gerald dies. David refuses to have anything to do with Gerald's body and the body goes to the county morgue. It will sit there a year and then be cremated–the ashes buried in a mass grave with all the other hapless souls who will die this year.

Discussion Questions

- If David refused to make decisions about Gerald's treatment, who would?
- With David's history with Gerald, do you believe that he has the right to make the decision to stop life-sustaining treatment?

A patient *with* capacity has the right to make decisions about his or her own medical treatment. A patient who *lacks* capacity cannot make a decision. A surrogate decision-maker, absent an advance directive, must make the decision for the patient. A patient who lacks the capacity to make a specific decision may have capacity for designating a surrogate decision-maker.

If there is no advance directive and no earlier designation of a surrogate by a formerly well-capacitated patient, the common practice is to turn to a close family member. However, in California and some other states, there is no law requiring it. Unlike states that follow an intestate succession or next-of-kin mandate, California statutes require only that the surrogate is an adult. That is all that it says. The surrogate decision-maker does not need to be a family member or even a spouse, and in many cases, should not be either.[1]

We do not use a family member as a surrogate if there is an advance directive and the family member's decisions are in conflict with the patient's expressed wishes or fundamental best interests. In addition, due to circumstances that have changed since the patient designated the family member, such as divorce, there may be evidence that that individual would no longer be the patient's chosen surrogate decision-maker. Further, we cannot overlook the incapacity of a surrogate decision-maker. Finally, a family member may be either estranged or unable to let go.

When a patient has had a full opportunity to appoint a surrogate but has not selected a family member, then there is even less evidence that the family member should be the surrogate decision-maker. Typically, there will more evidence that the patient wants someone else to be the surrogate. For example, a patient may be in the emergency room because of trauma after a fall. She may be about to undergo emergency surgery. A family member is at her bedside. When the patient is asked who she wants as surrogate, she does not appoint the family member at the bedside. As such, that family member should not make decisions for the patient. Similarly, a son who states, "I don't care what you do with Mother. Whatever my sister wants, I want the opposite," should obviously not be a surrogate decision-maker.

A patient does not lack for a surrogate decision-maker just because she has no spouse or next-of-kin. In many cases, an unconventional surrogate decision-maker might be best. An unconventional surrogate who knows the patient well may make better decisions for the patient than next-of-kin. This unconventional surrogate may be a close friend, a live-in companion who is not married to the patient, a significant other not married to the patient, a long-time neighbor, the patient's clergy, or the director of the homeless shelter that the patient frequents. The most appropriate surrogate for the patient is someone who has loving and intimate knowledge of the patient's values. In some cases, family members have only remote knowledge of the patient's values or are outright estranged. An unconventional surrogate might better represent the patient's most fully developed value system. (Surrogate decision-making committees will be addressed below.)

Above all, surrogate decision-making laws and policies should not hinder the patient's ability to die naturally and comfortably. An incapacitated patient does not need to be condemned to life-sustaining technology that she would not want.[2] This principle should apply in all settings, including hospitals, skilled nursing facilities, and homes. The rationale is that most people would prefer a natural death to a prolonged or painful dying process. There is generally no evidence that an incapacitated patient would want something that the surrogate decision-maker would not want for him or herself.

There are two standards for surrogate decision-making. The first is substituted judgment, in which the surrogate "stands in the shoes" of the patient. A decision made according to substituted judgment is the *exact* decision that the patient would made if she could. The substituted judgment standard is rare. It involves more than knowing the patient's values, attitudes about sickness, suffering, and medical treatment, and death. [3]

Unfortunately, knowing for a fact exactly what the patient would want in the specific situation is rare. Under the substituted judgment standard, it is not sufficient just to know and love the patient. The surrogate must have previously spoken about the exact circumstances and obtained the patient's exact decision. Subsequently, we can see why the use of the substituted judgment standard is rare. Most so-called substituted judgments are actually opinions about the patient's best interests.

Difficulties with substituted judgment have to do with the evidence and clarity of preferences:

- Determinate statements have the greatest evidentiary weight: "I would not want to be kept on a ventilator if I were in a persistent vegetative state." This evidentiary weight is probably required for the clear and convincing evidence standard in substituted judgment cases like Cruzan v. Director. Statements such as: "I don't want to be kept alive on machines," have less evidentiary weight because they lack the specificity of the previous statement.

- The more direct the statement, the greater its evidentiary weight: "I would not want to be kept alive on machines," versus a statement made at a family funeral: "Aunt Martha should not have been kept alive on machines."

- Of course, the greater the number of sources for the evidence, the greater its evidentiary weight, just as a more a reliable witness produces greater evidentiary weight.

- Finally, repeated statements given over a long period have greater evidentiary weight than two statements made in a short period, as they must represent the patient's established value system. [4]

It appears that surrogates generally predict patients' actual preferences about life-sustaining treatment only slightly better than chance. Therefore, we must consider whether the patient has a stronger interest in the identity of the surrogate than in how a decision is made.[5] A patient may not have strong beliefs about whether to choose or refuse life-sustaining treatment but may have confidence that the surrogate will make the correct decisions. Many elderly patients care more about family consensus than they care about what decisions are made.

When an incapacitated patient has not indicated preferences about medical care, the surrogate's decisions should be based upon the "best-interests" of the patient. In actual practice, most so-called substituted judgments are really best-interests cases. Under the best-interests standard, the surrogate's decisions should be the same as a reasonable adult would make if faced with the same circumstances. (Contrast this with the informed consent standards, where we care less about what the reasonable patient would choose and more about how a specific patient actually chose.) Most people do not want to live permanently in a vegetative state or die a prolonged death on life-sustaining treatment. In a decision about medical treatment, the surrogate should consider the relief of suffering, the patient's medical condition, and her quality of life.[6] The best interests of a patient are not necessarily preserving her biological life at all costs.

A surrogate decision-maker, using the best-interests standard to decide about a treatment, is in effect deciding whether the treatment is ordinary or extraordinary. The surrogate may consider factors such as the financial, physical, emotional, and moral burdens to the family caregivers if the patient survives. The patient's *manufactured disability*–a result of long-time survival on life-sustaining treatment–exacts a toll on the family and on the community.[7] If there is a cost to the community–an inequitable allocation of a scarce resource–such as a bed in an intensive care unit–the resource must be transferred to the patient who will survive the hospital admission.

Sometimes, we have *some* evidence of the patient's wishes but not enough to use substituted judgment. In these cases, an intermediate standard may be used.

We consider only the best interests of the specific patient. What might be in the best interests of one patient may not be the best interests of another patient, even under the same medical circumstances. What is at issue is the *relationship* between the patient's medical condition and her quality of life. This means that a surrogate cannot, while making a decision for the specific patient, refuse treatment that is considered ordinary. However, the surrogate can refuse treatment that is extraordinary, based on the patient's own values and the quality of life that would be acceptable to her. When the patient's medical condition leaves the patient without a quality of life that she would tolerate, then the biological life of the patient can be let go.

In other cases, a patient may have recovered (albeit perhaps below her baseline medical condition) from serious illnesses in the past. The family may decide that the patient is a "fighter" and the present illness is just one more from which the patient will recover and based upon this irrational certainty they want "everything possible" to be done.

There are exceptional circumstances in which legal counsel should be consulted if a decision to withdraw or withhold treatment is likely to result in the death of the patient. Such situations arise when the patient's condition is the result of a suspected criminal action or if the patient's condition was created or aggravated by a medical accident.

Case 7-2. Dementia and the Ventilator.

Lois Green is an eighty-five-year-old patient with dementia. She is alert but very confused. She knows her name but not her situation. Lois develops aspiration pneumonia because she choked on water. Lois receives ventilator support and a gastrostomy tube for feeding. She cannot be weaned from the ventilator and, after a week, she receives a tracheostomy. Lois lacks decision-making capacity but, when asked, she also indicates that she wants to stay on the ventilator. The hospital case manager applies for Medicaid on Lois's behalf and is

searching for a sub-acute facility that would take a long-term ventilator patient.

Lois has an advance directive naming her sister as her agent, but her sister died several years ago. Lois has no remaining family. She does have a friend of fifty years, Anne, who visits her daily and advocates for Lois. Anne maintains that Lois does not know what the ventilator is. She states that Lois would never want to live the way she is living if she understood the situation. She vehemently states that Lois never would have wanted to live on a ventilator and would never have agreed to artificial nutrition. Anne is not a legally designated agent but qualifies as a surrogate decision-maker because she knows and loves Lois and has her best interests at heart.

Lois's primary care physician agrees with Anne's decision. However, the attending physician is reluctant to withdraw the ventilator as Lois had indicated that she did not want it removed. Lois's primary care physician points out that Lois does not have capacity to make the decision to live on the ventilator. Anne is certain that Lois would not want to live tied to life-sustaining treatment and would prefer to be let go. The ethics consultant recommends, in accordance with Anne's knowledge of and love for Lois, that the ventilator and feeding tube should be withdrawn.

Discussion Questions

- Does Lois have the capacity to consent to life-sustaining treatment? Does she have the capacity to refuse it?
- Lois never made a decision about life-sustaining treatment. Do you believe Anne when she states that Lois would rather be allowed to die?

- Does the fact that many previously "independent" persons learn to live with dependence on life-sustaining treatment and enjoy their lives affect whether Lois should be allowed to die?

Chapter 8. Advance Directives and Physician Orders for Life-Sustaining Treatment (POLST)

Advance Directives

Case 8-1. The Advance Directive.

Norma Jenkins is a sixty-five-year-old woman with severe narrowing of her left carotid artery. Because of the high risk of a debilitating stroke, her physician recommends surgery to correct the narrowing. He informs Norma that the surgery has a small risk of a cerebral vascular accident (CVA or stroke). When Norma and her physician are discussing the risks and benefits of the treatment and how it might promote her quality of life, both Norma and her physician review her advance directive. As executed, it states:

> √ (a) Choice NOT to Prolong Life
>
> I do not want my life to be prolonged if:
>
>> (1) I have an incurable and irreversible condition that will result in my death within a relatively short time,
>>
>> (2) I become unconscious and, to a reasonable degree of medical certainty, I will not regain consciousness, or
>>
>> (3) the likely risks and burdens of treatment would outweigh the expected benefits.

Norma's late husband was appointed as agent. Norma does not want to complete a new advance directive as she does not believe that she has anyone who could act as decision-maker.

Norma's surgery is successful but shortly afterward, she experiences a stroke. Norma is taken back to the operating room and a large clot is removed. Norma continues to exhibit signs of a severe stroke, including paralysis, loss of consciousness, unreactive pupils, and responsiveness only to painful stimuli. Over the following week, Norma's condition does not improve. She requires a ventilator but then develops a ventilator-associated pneumonia.

Norma's physician asks for a neurology consultation. The neurologists indicate that it could take several months before Norma's prognosis could be certain. They feel that there is:

- A three percent chance that she can recover most of her mental and physical capacity. They decline to explain "most."

- A thirty-five percent chance that she will die without recovering consciousness.

- A sixty percent chance that Norma will recover but be cognitively damaged and probably bed-bound.

- An eighty percent chance that Norma will need assisted nutrition and hydration.

Norma's physician is unsure about how to interpret the patient's advance directive in light of this prognosis. Finally, he decides that the three percent chance of "most" of her physical and mental capacity is not good enough. That medical condition would not promote for Norma a quality of life that she would accept. He writes the order and withdraws the ventilator. Norma dies a day afterward.

Discussion Questions

- **Does Norma's advance directive sufficiently guide her physician's decision given the chances of various outcomes?**

- **How might Norma's advance directive be revised to express her wishes regarding the various possible outcomes?**

An advance directive is a legal document that provides an opportunity for a patient to plan for future medical treatment in the event that he loses decision-making capacity either temporarily or permanently. It allows a patient with capacity to articulate preferences regarding medical treatment, including life-sustaining treatment. Optimally, the patient's preferences are discussed with family or other loved ones as well as the physician.

The Federal Patient Self-Determination Act of 1991 requires that upon admission, hospital-admitting personnel must ask if the patient has an advance directive. If the patient has an advance directive, the admitting worker requests a copy. If the patient does not have an advance directive, the worker asks if the patient wants to execute one. Clinical social workers or chaplains usually provide explanations of advance directive forms to facilitate viable patient decision-making.

It is first important to note that the absence of an advance directive does not mean that the patient wants aggressive treatment. Likewise, the presence of an advance directive does not mean that the patient should automatically have a Do-Not-Resuscitate (DNR) order. The physician needs to actually read the advance directive in order to determine the patient's preferences.

A patient's family may not override an advance directive if it contains clear and unambiguous instructions. However, most advance directive forms are not specific enough to allow a surrogate to withdraw or withhold treatment that is ordinary and in the best interests of the patient.

An advance directive is comprised of two parts. The first part is the appointment of an agent (or agents) to make healthcare decisions when the person lacks capacity to make treatment decisions for him or herself. This part is called a durable power of attorney for healthcare–*durable* used here indicates that the directive survives the patient's incapacity. The second part is a description of the kind of medical treatment the patient wants or does not want when facing serious illness. This is now called a healthcare treatment directive, previously known commonly as a living will.

Most standardized advance directive forms are quite limited in the conditions that they cover and the subsequent decisions that need to be made. Advance directives generally provide instructions that apply only if the patient is in a terminal condition or permanently unconscious. However, the majority of health care decisions that need to be made for patients lacking capacity concern discharge and placement options, as well as treatment options short of withdrawing or withholding life-sustaining treatment.

(2.1) END-OF-LIFE DECISIONS: I direct that my health care providers and others involved in my care provide, withhold, or withdraw treatment in accordance with the choice I have marked below:

    ☐ (a) Choice Not to Prolong Life

    I do not want my life to be prolonged if (1) I have an incurable and irreversible condition that will result in my death within a relatively short time, (2) I become unconscious and, to a reasonable degree of medical certainty, I will not regain consciousness, or (3) the likely risks and burdens of treatment would outweigh the expected benefits, OR

    ☐ (b) Choice to Prolong Life

    I want my life to be prolonged as long as possible within the limits of generally accepted health care standards.

(2.2) RELIEF FROM PAIN: Except as I state in the following space, I direct that treatment for alleviation of pain or discomfort be provided at all times, even if it hastens my death:

The biggest issue encountered here is that the instructions in most advance directive forms are generally either too vague or too specific. For instance, among the terms that are too vague, we find: "relatively short time." Does that mean six hours? One day? Two days? A week, a month? Also, far too vague is the phrase "to a reasonable degree of medical certainty." Is that five percent? 85%? 99.9999%? Finally, we have: "the risks and burdens of treatment would outweigh the expected benefits." This is, while very common, just too nebulous and is essentially meaningless to most people.

Among the terms that are too specific, we may highlight: "incurable and irreversible condition." Not all conditions for which a patient might want to limit aggressive treatment occur when the patient's condition is incurable or irreversible. Life-and-death decisions may have to be made before or during a surgical procedure, for example, from which the patient has a moderate chance of surviving. In addition, advance directives do not generally cover conditions such as dementia, where people may want to refuse treatments altogether.

Because of both the vagueness and over specificity of the healthcare treatment directive, the most important part of the advance directive is the appointment of an agent to interpret the treatment directive and to make the right decisions. The second most important part of the advance directive is the conversation that the patient has with said agent. William H. Colby makes this point: "I don't believe that I can anticipate all of the maladies that might befall me or the potential treatments that might or might not help. More importantly, a written living will cannot advocate for me. I want a breathing, reasoning advocate, one who understands everything [I have said]."[1]

Having an advance directive limiting life-sustaining treatment will not prevent a patient from having cardiopulmonary resuscitation (CPR) if his heart stops or if he stops breathing. The advance directive is not a physician order. It must be translated into physician orders. Even in an advance directive with the "Choice Not to Prolong Life," a patient may receive CPR unless and until a Do-Not-Resuscitate order (DNR) is written and signed by a physician. Without a DNR, the default position for most hospitals is to perform CPR.

Because advance directives must be translated into physician orders, a physician might sign orders inconsistent with the patient's advance directive. By law, healthcare providers must follow the instructions in the healthcare treatment part of an advance directive as interpreted by the agent. Realistically, however, a physician might sign orders that are inconsistent with an advance directive. In this case, there is no practical recourse for the patient or his agent other than to contact the ethics committee.[2]

A healthcare provider must comply with an agent's decision unless it would require medically ineffective treatment. Healthcare providers have both legal and ethical duties to respect advance directives. However, should an agent demand medically ineffective treatment, the healthcare providers' duties to comply come to an end.

The California Probate Code Section 4735, and similar laws of other states, codifies this:

> A health care provider or health care institution may decline to comply with an individual health care instruction or health care decision that requires medically ineffective health care or health care contrary to generally accepted health care standards applicable to the health care provider or institution.

A medical center that refuses to implement a healthcare decision requiring medically ineffective treatment, or that is against hospital policy, must facilitate the transfer of the patient to another healthcare institution that is willing to comply with the decision.

Realistically, again, if a patient's family members oppose the instructions of the advance directive agent, the advance directive may not be honored. Likewise, a physician may disagree with an advance directive that limits life-sustaining treatment and not honor it. The agent may then be forced to contact the ethics committee. This is why patients executing advance directives must appoint agents who can be relied on to fight for their instructions.

An advance directive may be revoked by the patient at any time, either verbally or in writing. If the revocation is in writing, the patient should cross out the pages of the advance directive and sign his name on the lines. Advance directives need to be either witnessed or notarized, and this is the point at which they generally fail in an emergency. Most hospitals do not have a notary on staff and 24-hour mobile notaries are very expensive. An employee of the medical center, a physician, or a nurse cannot witness a patient's advance directive. For example, in the California advance directive form, one of the witnesses must sign a statement that he is not related to the patient in any way and is not entitled to any part of the patient's estate. This means that in an emergency, in the middle of the night, an authorized witness may not be readily found. Desperate healthcare providers have been known to use the family members of another patient as witnesses in an emergency.

Moving on, we will note that most state's probate codes allow that a healthcare provider may refuse to comply with a healthcare instruction for reasons of conscience.

The "Five Wishes" form is friendlier—but is not held as a legal advance directive in many states. Five Wishes has some advantages, however. It is also slightly less vague and slightly more specific than an advance directive. The Five Wishes form is more emotionally based, more "touchy-feely." It is not a statutory advance directive, but it is good written evidence of the patient's preferences in the absence of an advance directive.

Many specialized advance directive forms exist to assist patients with special needs. *Thinking Ahead* is an advance directive designed for patients with intellectual disabilities. Videos are available to help the intellectually disabled patient fill out the form. There are advance directive forms with pictures and simple language to assist patients with low health literacy to make their wishes known. Psychiatric advance directives may be completed by a mentally ill patient whose decision-making capacity is episodic. The patient fills out the psychiatric advance directive with his psychiatrist when he is in a "cool moment"; the psychiatric advance directive then takes effect when the patient lacks coherence and insight into his condition and refuses treatment. Many different religious authorities have designed advance directives that comply with their traditions, including a Halachic living will, a Christian Science advance directive, and a living will for followers of Amitabha Buddha.

Physician Orders for Life-Sustaining Treatment (POLST)

Case 8-2. Physician Orders for Life-Sustaining Treatment.

Herman Jessup, a seventy-one-year-old man with chronic obstructive pulmonary disease, is recovering in a skilled nursing facility following a bout of pneumonia. Herman's physician tells him that he will probably experience an inability to breathe sometime in the next year. She explains that CPR will almost

certainly not work. Herman's physician further explains that even if CPR restarts Herman's heart, he would require a ventilator. The physician states—quite strongly—that Herman would eventually die on the ventilator unless he makes another decision now.

Herman states that he does not want CPR to even be attempted, as he has no intention of dying in an intensive care unit on a ventilator. His physician writes an out-of-hospital Do-Not-Resuscitate (DNR) order in his chart at the nursing home.

A week later, Herman develops increasing shortness of breath and decreasing responsiveness. The nursing home staff call for the paramedics. Although Herman had asked his physician to write a DNR, he does not have a POLST. The nursing home staff cannot find the out-of-hospital DNR. The paramedics attempt CPR. Herman is transferred to the emergency room at the local hospital. Without a POLST, the emergency physician's order is: "Full code for now. We'll think about it later." After intubating and sedating Herman in the emergency room, he is transferred to the intensive care unit where he dies one week later after an attempt at resuscitation that lasts twenty-five minutes.

Discussion Questions
- What happened? How did Herman end up dying a death that he plainly did not wish to endure?
- Why, after the CPR was performed, did Herman end up in the intensive care unit against his wishes?
- Why would the paramedics not have a protocol that would enable them to follow an out-of-hospital DNR?

Physician Orders for Life-Sustaining Treatment, or POLST, is a form signed both by the patient or surrogate and by the physician.

POLST is a set of immediately actionable, signed medical orders on brightly colored card stock in a standard shade. POLST is a one page, check-the-box form. Not all states have POLST but those who do have a standard state form. As of the writing of this book, approximately half of the states in the United States have check-the-box forms very similar to POLST, although they may be called by different names. For example, Colorado's form is called MOST, or Medical Orders for Scope of Treatment.

HIPAA PERMITS DISCLOSURE OF POLST TO OTHER HEALTH CARE PROVIDERS AS NECESSARY

Physician Orders for Life-Sustaining Treatment (POLST)

EMSA #111 B
(Effective 1/1/2016)*

First follow these orders, then contact **Physician/NP/PA**. A copy of the signed POLST form is a legally valid physician order. Any section not completed implies full treatment for that section. POLST complements an Advance Directive and is not intended to replace that document.

Patient Last Name:	Date Form Prepared:
Patient First Name:	Patient Date of Birth:
Patient Middle Name:	Medical Record # (optional)

A
Check One

CARDIOPULMONARY RESUSCITATION (CPR): *If patient has no pulse and is not breathing.*
If patient is NOT in cardiopulmonary arrest, follow orders in Sections B and C.

☐ Attempt Resuscitation/CPR (Selecting CPR in Section A <u>requires</u> selecting Full Treatment in Section B)
☐ Do Not Attempt Resuscitation/DNR (Allow Natural Death)

B
Check One

MEDICAL INTERVENTIONS: *If patient is found with a pulse and/or is breathing.*

☐ <u>Full Treatment</u> – primary goal of prolonging life by all medically effective means.
In addition to treatment described in Selective Treatment and Comfort-Focused Treatment, use intubation, advanced airway interventions, mechanical ventilation, and cardioversion as indicated.
☐ *Trial Period of Full Treatment.*

☐ <u>Selective Treatment</u> – goal of treating medical conditions while avoiding burdensome measures.
In addition to treatment described in Comfort-Focused Treatment, use medical treatment, IV antibiotics, and IV fluids as indicated. Do not intubate. May use non-invasive positive airway pressure. Generally avoid intensive care.
☐ *Request transfer to hospital only if comfort needs cannot be met in current location.*

☐ <u>Comfort-Focused Treatment</u> – primary goal of maximizing comfort.
Relieve pain and suffering with medication by any route as needed; use oxygen, suctioning, and manual treatment of airway obstruction. Do not use treatments listed in Full and Selective Treatment unless consistent with comfort goal. Request transfer to hospital only if comfort needs cannot be met in current location.

Additional Orders: _____

C
Check One

ARTIFICIALLY ADMINISTERED NUTRITION: *Offer food by mouth if feasible and desired.*

☐ Long-term artificial nutrition, including feeding tubes.   Additional Orders: _____
☐ Trial period of artificial nutrition, including feeding tubes. _____
☐ No artificial means of nutrition, including feeding tubes. _____

D

INFORMATION AND SIGNATURES:

Discussed with: ☐ Patient (Patient Has Capacity)   ☐ Legally Recognized Decisionmaker

☐ Advance Directive dated _____, available and reviewed →   Health Care Agent if named in Advance Directive:
☐ Advance Directive not available   Name: _____
☐ No Advance Directive   Phone: _____

Signature of Physician / Nurse Practitioner / Physician Assistant (Physician/NP/PA)
My signature below indicates to the best of my knowledge that these orders are consistent with the patient's medical condition and preferences.

| Print Physician/NP/PA Name: | Physician/NP/PA Phone #: | Physician/PA License #, NP Cert. #: |
| Physician/NP/PA Signature: *(required)* | | Date: |

Signature of Patient or Legally Recognized Decisionmaker
I am aware that this form is voluntary. By signing this form, the legally recognized decisionmaker acknowledges that this request regarding resuscitative measures is consistent with the known desires of, and with the best interest of, the individual who is the subject of the form.

Print Name:		Relationship: *(write self if patient)*
Signature: *(required)*	Date:	**FOR REGISTRY USE ONLY**
Mailing Address (street/city/state/zip):	Phone Number:	

SEND FORM WITH PATIENT WHENEVER TRANSFERRED OR DISCHARGED
*Form versions with effective dates of 1/1/2009, 4/1/2011 or 10/1/2014 are also valid

Unlike an advance directive, POLST is a physician order. Its standardized form makes it easy to interpret in an instant and makes it easy to transport across healthcare settings.

Legally and ethically, honoring a POLST is mandatory, just as honoring an advance directive is mandatory. However, unlike an advance directive, POLST both expresses the patient's values *and* is a physician order to provide or not provide life-sustaining treatment. This is why both the patient (or his agent or surrogate) and the patient's physician must sign the document.

POLST gives the patient more control over his end-of-life care by specifying the types of medical treatment he wants or abjures. The POLST form orders healthcare providers to provide the treatments that the patient wants and avoid those that he does not want.

POLST provides direction for a range of end-of-life medical treatments:

- Cardiopulmonary resuscitations (CPR)
- Intermediate treatments such as positive airway devices
- Gastrostomy or feeding tubes
- Comfort care

POLST addresses a range of life-sustaining interventions as well as the preferred intensity of treatment for each intervention.

The POLST form is recognized, adopted, and honored across all treatment settings. All healthcare providers, including first responders, must legally follow POLST orders, if known, except if the treatment is medically ineffective or contrary to the standard of care in the community. POLST is a portable document that transfers with the patient across all settings within a given state:

- Assisted living facilities
- Clinics
- Emergency medical systems
- Home health and hospice
- Skilled nursing facilities
- Hospitals

Because POLST is transportable, healthcare providers must honor POLST even if the signatory physician does not have admitting privileges at the facility to which the patient is being admitted.

POLST is designed for people who have a chronic progressive illness on a downward trajectory, a terminal illness, or are medically frail. Most patients with POLSTs have a prognosis of one year of life or less. Nursing home residents and hospice patients use POLST, though POLST is also used by any medically frail or terminally ill patients. POLST experts say: "We ask doctors to ask themselves: "Would I be surprised if this patient died in the next year?" If the answer is no, then we recommend that the physician have a discussion about end-of-life treatment preferences and work with the patient to see that a POLST form is completed."

As with an advance directive, the most important part of a POLST is the conversation it memorializes between the patient and her physician.

The problem with an advance directive is that when a debilitated patient in crisis is rescued by the paramedics and arrives in the emergency room, no one has time to interpret the patient's advance directive. This is why so many patients with advance directives limiting life-sustaining treatment are given CPR and end up intubated in the intensive care unit against their will. A physician in Oregon, where POLST originated, stated: "[Paramedics] are sick and tired of breaking the ribs on a 90-year-old woman who weighs 80 pounds. They think it's wonderful that they don't have to attempt resuscitation on people they will fail to help and who don't want CPR."

Again, we see that advance directives are usually too vague or too specific. A patient's wishes about a specific treatment are often not apparent. In addition, advance directives are not always clearly defined and must be translated into physician orders. This means that there may often be a lag time between the medical center having a copy of the patient's advance directive and the physician actually writing consistent orders. POLST is an *already* actionable medical order that is easy to access and easy to understand across a wide array of circumstances.

As POLST is a physician order, it must be signed by both the physician and the patient. It can be signed by the patient's decision-maker if the patient lacks capacity. In contrast, an advance directive cannot be signed by a surrogate decision-maker. However, it is preferable to have an advance directive executed prior to the POLST so that the agent named in the advance directive can sign the POLST.

While a POLST is transferrable and honored across all health care settings, the DNR order is a strictly medical order that is not honored outside the hospital (and often not even honored for subsequent admissions to the same hospital). As such DNR orders need to be renewed in every setting, again and again. A POLST includes a DNR but has several advantages over a DNR. Both the POLST and the DNR are physician orders and both preclude CPR if the patient is not breathing and his heart is not beating. Both are appropriate for the medically frail or those with chronic or serious illness.

However, POLST is considerably more comprehensive than the standard Do-Not-Resuscitate form. POLST allows for choosing resuscitation, as well as refusing it, and allows for decisions about other important medical treatments, such as artificial nutrition. In addition, POLST does not permit a chemical code order. A chemical code is CPR without chest compressions and electric shock; only medications are used. However, if the patient's heart has stopped, the patient has no circulation and the medications do not go anywhere. Chemical codes are generally considered unethical.

A POLST should be revisited every time that the patient is transferred to a new health care facility or if the patient's prognosis changes significantly. A POLST form can be revoked either verbally or in writing. If a patient wishes to revoke a POLST, he need only execute another POLST with a later date. It is very important to date the POLST form so that the most recent version can easily be identified in the case of conflicting documents. If a patient lacks capacity, the agent named in the patient's advance directive normally should sign the POLST. If the patient has a POLST but no advance directive, then his choice of surrogate decision-maker may be documented in his medical chart.

A	CARDIOPULMONARY RESUSCITATION (CPR): *If patient has no pulse and is not breathing.*
Check One	*If patient is NOT in cardiopulmonary arrest, follow orders in Sections B and C.*
	☐ Attempt Resuscitation/CPR (Selecting CPR in Section A requires selecting Full Treatment in Section B)
	☐ Do Not Attempt Resuscitation/DNR (Allow Natural Death)

Section A of the POLST addresses events such as acute myocardial infarction (AMI), or heart attack.

96

B	**MEDICAL INTERVENTIONS:**	*If patient is found with a pulse and/or is breathing.*

Check One

☐ **Full Treatment** – **primary goal of prolonging life by all medically effective means.**
In addition to treatment described in Selective Treatment and Comfort-Focused Treatment, use intubation, advanced airway interventions, mechanical ventilation, and cardioversion as indicated.
    ☐ *Trial Period of Full Treatment.*

☐ **Selective Treatment** – **goal of treating medical conditions while avoiding burdensome measures.**
In addition to treatment described in Comfort-Focused Treatment, use medical treatment, IV antibiotics, and IV fluids as indicated. Do not intubate. May use non-invasive positive airway pressure. Generally avoid intensive care.
    ☐ *Request transfer to hospital only if comfort needs cannot be met in current location.*

☐ **Comfort-Focused Treatment** – **primary goal of maximizing comfort.**
Relieve pain and suffering with medication by any route as needed; use oxygen, suctioning, and manual treatment of airway obstruction. Do not use treatments listed in Full and Selective Treatment unless consistent with comfort goal. *Request transfer to hospital only if comfort needs cannot be met in current location.*

Additional Orders: _____

Section B of the POLST addresses treatments such as intubation, as opposed to comfort care. The goal of *Full Treatment* is to prolong life by all medically effective treatments. The goal of *Selective Treatment* is to provide beneficial and not burdensome treatments. The goal of *Comfort-Focused Treatment* is to maximize comfort. Note that comfort-focused treatment must be provided no matter what level of treatment the patient selects.

C	**ARTIFICIALLY ADMINISTERED NUTRITION:**	*Offer food by mouth if feasible and desired.*

Check One

☐ Long-term artificial nutrition, including feeding tubes.   Additional Orders: _____
☐ Trial period of artificial nutrition, including feeding tubes. _____
☐ No artificial means of nutrition, including feeding tubes. _____

Section C of the POLST addresses artificial nutrition and hydration in the event of a cerebral vascular accident (CVA), or a stroke.

In Section A, note that choosing "Attempt Resuscitation/CPR" requires selecting full treatment in Section B. CPR is defined to include chest compressions and Advanced Cardiac Life Support Procedures, including intubation. If CPR is desired, then the full array of resuscitation procedures will be implemented. This means that if CPR is successful initially and the heart is revived, then it is extremely likely that the patient will end up on a ventilator. A patient not willing to accept the full panoply of procedures, including ventilator treatment, should not have CPR performed.

Depending on the POLST form, a patient should be able to select a DNR in Section A, and the "Full Treatment" option in Section B. Section A specifically applies when there is full cardiac and respiratory distress and Section B specifically applies when the patient has a pulse and is breathing. Subsequently, Section A does not apply where there is no cardiac arrest and Section B does not apply when there is cardiac arrest.

In Section B, a patient may choose to write in a "trial period." Then, if the patient's health is failing and the patient requires long-term ventilator support, ventilator treatments could be withdrawn, and the patient will be allowed to die. If a patient chooses "Full Treatment" in Section B, we must consider asking the patient what should be done if the full, aggressive treatment is not working and her physician believes that she will not recover.

In Section B, "Selective Treatment" is without question the most complex category of treatment choices to understand. Patients choosing this category generally are asking not to be treated with invasive medical procedures such as mechanical ventilation or to undergo major surgery such as open-heart surgery. However, intensive care unit treatment is not strictly prohibited. For instance, a patient who has chosen "Selective Treatment" could be treated in the intensive care unit for a limited period of time. Patients who choose "Selective Treatment" do not want aggressive treatments that have a low chance of success and could lead to further debility.

It's important to note that Section B requires that "Comfort-Focused Treatment" be included in "Full Treatment" and "Selective Treatment."

Section C addresses the eventualities for types of events like a cerebral vascular accident, a stroke. Some patients may not want to live after a major stroke that leaves them completely dependent on others and therefore would not want artificial nutrition and hydration. A patient may wish for gastrostomy treatment to be initiated but not continued if the chances of recovery are uncertain or poor. A patient may even add explanations and exclusions under "Additional Orders" in Section B. A time-limited "Trial Period" may be required before we know if the course of treatment is effective.

The reverse side of the POLST form provides additional information and interpretation of the orders.

Using POLST

- Any incomplete section of POLST implies full treatment for that section.

Section A:
- If found pulseless and not breathing, no defibrillator (including automated external defibrillators) or chest compressions should be used on a patient who has chosen "Do Not Attempt Resuscitation."

Section B:
- When comfort cannot be achieved in the current setting, the patient, including someone with "Comfort-Focused Treatment," should be transferred to a setting able to provide comfort (e.g., treatment of a hip fracture).
- Non-invasive positive airway pressure includes continuous positive airway pressure (CPAP), bi-level positive airway pressure (BiPAP), and bag valve mask (BVM) assisted respirations.
- IV antibiotics and hydration generally are not "Comfort-Focused Treatment."
- Treatment of dehydration prolongs life. If a patient desires IV fluids, indicate "Selective Treatment" or "Full Treatment."
- Depending on local EMS protocol, "Additional Orders" written in Section B may not be implemented by EMS personnel.

It states that intravenous antibiotics and hydration are generally not considered "Comfort-Focused Treatment," because treatment of dehydration either prolongs life or causes fluid overload at the end of life; if the patient desires intravenous fluids, the POLST must indicate "Selective Treatment" or "Full Treatment." Honoring a POLST is mandatory in most states, including California.

In 2010, Emily DeArmond, who suffered from multiple, severe medical conditions and who was cared for by her mother, Julie, suffered a swift decline. She was taken to Kaiser Anaheim Medical Center, of which she was a member. Emily had a POLST designating *Limited Interventions*, and selected *No Intubation* in Section B. In the emergency department, a physician reportedly refused to review the POLST and subsequently intubated Emily against her mother's entreaties. At her mother's request, Emily was transferred to another Kaiser facility, was extubated, and died the next day. In 2011, Julie DeArmond filed a complaint against Kaiser Permanente claiming that the physician caused her and Emily's distress. Kaiser was also named because of its lack of training on POLST. Julie contended that the physician and Kaiser caused intentional infliction of emotional distress to both Emily and Julie. *Julie DeArmond v. Permanente Medical Group (2011)*. The case was settled.

Chapter 9. Futility

Case 9-1. Using New, Expensive Drugs.

Jack White is eighty-six years old. One night, Jack is transferred by ambulance from a skilled nursing facility where he lives to the small, local community hospital because he is unresponsive and short of breath. He is diagnosed with a cerebral hemorrhage, respiratory failure, pneumonia, and hypotension. He also has end-stage dementia, insulin-dependent diabetes, congestive heart failure, and several wounds on his buttocks. Jack's family wants "everything done" and specifically mentions a new drug. They ask the physicians at the community hospital for that drug, but the pharmacy formulary does not include it. The hospital therefore sends Jack by ambulance to the nearest facility that is able to administer the drug.

The intensivist at the regional, tertiary referral center is obligated to accept patients from the small, local hospital. On arrival, Jack is paralyzed on his right side, his eyes are unresponsive to light and he has a high white cell count, a raised temperature, and Gram-positive bacteria growing from two blood cultures.

Jack has been on three antibiotics for two days and is not improving. He requires mechanical ventilation and continuous infusion of vasopressors to maintain his blood pressure. He does not respond even to deeply painful stimuli. His family states that Jack is a "fighter" and repeat that they want "everything done."

Recent medical literature suggests that outcomes for patients with Jack's diagnoses improve following the administration of a recombinant factor medication. However, it is expensive and in short supply. It costs up to $8,000 per treatment course over 48 hours.

It is the opinion of the intensivist that, although the medication is one possible option, administering it to Jack would not improve his outcome. He believes that Jack is dying and the medication will not change the course of his illness, or, alternatively, Jack might lapse into a persistent vegetative state. However, Jack's primary physician reminds him that the family wants "everything done." He states that as such everything must be done until Jack's family changes their mind. He argues that "everything" means "everything possible." The intensivist disagrees and states that the definition of "everything" does not mean "everything possible," but "everything reasonable" and that the critical care team has the right to limit life-sustaining treatments, including expensive medications.

Discussion Questions

- Should we consider cost when we decide whether to give a gravely ill patient an expensive medication?
- Does Jack's family have the right to demand that Jack receive the medication if they pay for it themselves?

Those who call for the abandonment of the concept [of futility] have no substitute to offer. They persist in making decisions with, more or less, covert definitions. The common-sense notion that a time does come for all of us when death or disability exceeds our medical powers cannot be denied. This means that some operative way of making a decision when "enough is enough" is necessary. It is a mark of our mortality that we shall die. For each of us some determination of futility by any other name will become a reality. Some working definition therefore must be recognized by which the criterion of futility can be judged.[1]

The term *futile* is derived from the Latin word, *futilis,* a ceremonial vessel. A *futilis* has a rounded bottom with a hole in it. A *futilis* has no practical use. It is a purely ceremonial vessel. Therefore, futile treatment is "leaky."

The notion of medical futility is not a new concept. Although the Hippocratic treatises do not use the word "futility," they do state that physicians must "refuse to treat those overmastered by disease." The concept of futility recognizes that, at some point in each of our lives, we will be beyond medical rescue.

Some medical centers define futile treatment as "nonbeneficial" treatment. However, limiting the definition to benefit and burden is not sufficient. Futile medical treatment is always nonbeneficial. Nevertheless, telling a family that treatment is futile may be counter-productive. It may be softer—emotionally—to tell a family that a treatment is nonbeneficial. A distinction that does not change the status of the treatment but is, nevertheless, a more compassionate delivery.

At this point, we must consider that futile treatment is often inhumane treatment. "Overuse and underuse of care may occur simultaneously. For example, when futile efforts to cure are continued at the expense of efforts to relieve physical and psychological symptoms and help patients and families prepare emotionally, spiritually, and practically for death."[2]

The goal of medicine is not to extract every possible moment of biological life from a patient.

Recall our discussion about the goal of medicine. We said that a treatment may never be provided without a purpose; namely to promote the patient's values and her quality of life. *Medical treatments are not ends in themselves*–they are the skilled means of achieving noble goals. This means that a treatment is futile if it cannot accomplish its true goal: to promote the patient's values and quality of life.

Since one condition for determining that a treatment is futile is its repeated failure to fulfill the goal of treatment, it stands to reason that whether or not treatment is considered futile depends entirely upon how we define the goal. For example, asking a patient if she wants to be artificially ventilated for a limited period if she goes into respiratory failure identifies a treatment, *not* a goal. Artificial ventilation may not be futile if its use is compassionate. For example, the patient's goal may be to survive for three days so that a daughter in the military overseas may come to say good-bye. On the other hand, artificial ventilation may be futile if the patient is unlikely to survive long-term without the ventilator and she has no short-term imperative to fulfill. This means that until the goal has been understood and agreed upon, we cannot really determine whether or not a treatment is futile.

A futile treatment is any *indeterminate, long-term* medical treatment that, in the best judgment of medical professionals, meets one or more of the disjunctive conditions set forth below. By definition, futile treatment is indeterminate and long-term, thus time trials are excluded from this section and discussed afterwards.

Condition 1: A treatment is futile if it is medically ineffective.

Some bioethicists and physicians want to restrict the definition of futility to medically ineffective or physiological futility. For example, vasopressors do not successfully raise the blood pressure and prevent death. These bioethicists and physicians want to eliminate quality-of-life judgments and to make the definition of a futile treatment an empirical matter only to be decided by physicians. For example, the Society of Critical Care Medicine states that physiologically futile treatment is "value neutral."[3]

However, to specify physiological effectiveness as the goal of a treatment is not value-neutral; it is a value *judgment*. The goal of the treatment and the certainty needed to determine that it will be effective are value determinations. Even to determine prognosis is a value judgment. Most physicians have a tendency to overestimate prognosis, demonstrating in effect that many healthcare providers lean towards an optimistic outlook even (and sometimes especially) when and where optimism is just unwarranted. Even with prognostic indicators, physicians have been found to overestimate survival for critically ill patients by upwards of five times. In one study, physicians estimated that 1.1 percent of skilled nursing facility residents would die within six months - 71 percent actually died.[4] Physicians tend to overestimate prognosis for a variety of factors, including (but far from limited to): overconfidence in medical treatments, the belief that just one more treatment will fix everything, and perhaps most impactful - the natural tendency toward overconfidence in one's own skills.

David Crippen, a critical care physician, writes of his frustration because his specialty only considers medically ineffective treatment to be futile. "Patients may be stalled in suspended animation; they are not alive in the sense that we enjoy life but neither are they able to die as long as nutrition, hydration, ventilation, and perfusion are assured. In many cases reanimation of such patients is clearly impossible, even with the advanced medical technologies available to us."[5]

Condition 2: A treatment is futile if it produces medical effects but not medical benefits.

Futile treatment need not only be physiologically ineffective. As we have seen in the discussion of ordinary and extraordinary treatments, the goal of a medical treatment is more than preserving the patient's biological life and organ systems in the face of a fatal pathology. Remember, the goal of treatment is to benefit the patient as a whole. Therefore, a treatment may be considered futile if there is a good chance that it will have a specific effect on the patient's body but that the effect will not provide any benefit to the patient as a whole—body, intellect, emotion, and the overall totality of one's human experience.

Physicians are only obligated to offer treatments that have a reasonable chance of providing real benefits for the patient, regardless of whether they achieve effects. In addition, the determination of the balance of benefit and burden, so central to the distinction between ordinary and extraordinary treatment, is always to some degree a value judgment.

Condition 3: A treatment is futile if the patient's death is irreversibly imminent.

A treatment is futile if the physiological effect is achieved but the effect does not result in a significant duration of survival. The patient will die in the not-too-distant future from the fatal pathology that is being treated. When the patient's death is imminent, then any application of life-sustaining treatment will only prolong the moment and process of death. Determining when death is "imminent" is, of course, a value judgment. Does this mean that the patient will die within two weeks? Two days? Two hours?

Condition 4: A treatment is futile if the effect is irrelevant to the real condition of a dying patient.

A treatment is futile if it treats a secondary condition that will not postpone imminent death from the underlying fatal pathology that is the primary diagnosis. For example, it is futile to treat an actively dying cancer patient's pneumonia; conversely, "comfort" treatments are never to be considered futile, as their goal is in-line with easing the patient's suffering.

Pneumonia was once called "the old man's friend" because if left untreated, the patient slips away peacefully and with dignity in his sleep. When it is morally right to let a patient suffering from terminal cancer to die of pneumonia, we use nonsteroidal anti-inflammatory drugs (NSAIDs) and cooling measures for the fever, morphine or a similar drug, oxygen, repositioning for any shortness of breath, and benzodiazepines or other medications for anxiety and terminal agitation.

Condition 5: A treatment is futile if it will not end dependence on intensive medical treatment.

Any indeterminate, long-term treatment is futile when it is provided to a patient who has no realistic chance of surviving outside an acute care hospital. If a treatment has no reasonable chance of restoring the patient's health to a point that she can survive without life-sustaining treatment, it should be considered futile.[6] Contrast this with a situation where short-term treatment may have a nonmedical goal, such as allowing the patient to say good-bye to loved ones.

Condition 6: A treatment is futile if it cannot accomplish the patient's reasonable goals.

Nothing can be determined to be futile unless: (a) there is an express and recognizable goal; (b) there is a clear treatment plan aimed at achieving the goal; and (c) the goal cannot be reasonably expected to be achieved no matter how many times the treatment is repeated. A certain treatment may be futile in achieving one goal and not futile in achieving another.

A treatment is also futile if, statistically, it has little chance of being effective. Schneiderman proposes that a treatment is absolutely futile if it has a one percent chance of being effective. The choice of the acceptable risk level is, again, a value judgment - it might well be three percent or another number entirely. Schneiderman chooses one percent because it is within the statistical margin of error for determining the effectiveness of most life-sustaining treatments. Schneiderman states that his risk analysis is "quasi-numeric," therefore a quantitative condition, and not a purely qualitative metric. However, Schneiderman also admits that a treatment may be futile depending on the quality of the result that the treatment would produce, such as prolonging the biological life of a patient who is permanently unconscious. He treats the qualitative and quantitative conditions of futility as independent, meaning only one condition need be met for a physician to refuse to order the treatment. In short, a treatment is futile if it repeatedly fails to produce an intended effect. [7]

Under this condition, we do not treat one hundred patients with a "useless" treatment just to find an outlier. This means that a treatment is futile if it is highly improbable to be reliably effective. If a rare success cannot be predictably and systematically reproduced, then a statistical statement of probability is difficult. A treatment is considered useless depending upon the experiences of the physician and her colleagues, or reported empiric data.[8]

> If you truly want to make a case for attempting aggressive, life-sustaining, rib-cracking CPR on a patient who has a "one in a hundred chance" of recovering, you are claiming that it is appropriate to subject ninety-nine patients to an intervention that is painful, burdensome, and almost certainly useless in pursuit of one possible rare success. This violates medicine's duty to avoid imposing unnecessary suffering and the ethical duty of proportionality.[9]

Condition 7: A treatment is futile if it will cause harm or burden that outweighs any expected benefits.

Recalling the difference between ordinary and extraordinary treatment, a medical treatment is beneficial if it, for example, restores consciousness or maintains life where there is a reasonable hope of recovery. On the other hand, a medical treatment is burdensome if, for example, it results in excessive suffering for the patient or excessive expense for the family or the community. The risk of iatrogenic harm (side effects of medical care) from a treatment must also be considered. The balance of benefit and burden must always tip heavily toward burden for a treatment to be deemed futile.

Condition 8: A treatment is futile if it cannot reasonably be expected to be experienced by the patient as beneficial.

This is the most controversial condition as it rides squarely on a quality-of-life judgment. Under this condition, a treatment is futile it has no realistic chance of providing a benefit that the patient would ever have the capacity to recognize and appreciate. This condition means that the provision of indeterminate, long-term treatment, including artificial nutrition, hydration, and antibiotics to permanently unconscious or persistent vegetative-state patients, is futile because they cannot experience its benefits.

Since persistent vegetative patients will never experience the effects of artificial nutrition, the only benefit would be to allow time for them to recover consciousness. When they have been diagnosed, and this possibility has been excluded, then this life-sustaining treatment may be withheld or withdrawn.[10] We cannot justify the use of an expensive resource, such as a ventilator, for a permanently unconscious patient.[11] Most bioethicists agree that any treatment that merely preserves permanent unconsciousness is futile.

Condition 8 is less controversial when we recall that the determination of quality of life is made by the patient. Permanently unconscious or persistent vegetative-state patients have no quality of life. They enjoy no value other than mere biological life. We have said that when a patient has nothing more than a bare biological life, she can be let go. Thus, Condition 8 is a focused value judgment assessing the *absence* of quality of life.

Futile Treatment and the Standard of Care

Extraordinary treatment is optional. Futile treatment is not optional and should *never* be provided. Futile treatment is always contrary to generally accepted health care standards and is always contrary to the standard of care. Because futile treatment by definition never meets the standard of care, a physician commits malpractice when she provides it. Once a treatment has been found to be futile in a particular case, the physician(s) must withhold or withdraw it, despite the wishes of the patient and the patient's surrogate, and hospital policies should be written accordingly. Thus, futile treatment must never be offered to the patient or his decision-maker in the first place. There may be a virtually absolute negative right to refuse all life-sustaining treatment in the United States, but there is no corresponding positive right to demand futile treatment.[12]

Some patients and surrogates feel that the physician is abandoning them when the physician refuses to order futile life-sustaining treatment. However, we do not abandon patients even where treatment is futile; we accompany them to the end. While an over-treated death is feared, the opposite medical response—abandonment—is likewise frightening. Patients and those close to them may suffer physically and emotionally when physicians and nurses conclude that a patient is dying and then withdraw—passing by the hospital room on rounds, failing to follow up on the patient at home, and disregarding pain and other symptoms.[13] On the other hand—and make no mistake here—when we insist on continuing to provide burdensome, futile treatment we are actively condemning that patient to suffering.

In terms of individual treatments, cardiopulmonary resuscitation (CPR) is frequently futile.[14] CPR was developed for otherwise healthy individuals who experienced cardiac or respiratory distress during surgery or near-drowning. The American Medical Association estimates that CPR is attempted in nearly one-third of the two million deaths that occur in hospitals every year. This figure includes the frail, elderly, and other seriously ill patients. Treatments like CPR on a dying metastatic cancer patient simply will not work for long, if at all, and cause unnecessary and immense suffering at the end of life, namely rib fractures and increased respiratory secretions.

The default position for most hospitals is to attempt cardiopulmonary resuscitation. Without a Do-Not-Resuscitate (DNR) order in place, every patient in most medical centers is by default a full code, meaning she will receive CPR until minutes pass and it is not effective. "The words "full code" are not always written in the medical chart; the full code is simply a fact of hospital life."[15] Cardiopulmonary resuscitation is *violent*: chest compressions break ribs; forced intubation damages mouths and tracheas; electrical defibrillation burns the skin.

CPR is effective for some patients: for example, otherwise healthy patients who experience cardiac arrest during anesthesia. However, it does not work for sick patients with terminal cancer or the frail elderly. Most of these survivors live only a few more hours and sustain considerable anoxic neurological damage. Rarely do survivors return to baseline—the level of functioning that they had prior to arrest.

All things considered, CPR is *not fundamentally effective*. Further, taken as an observer, it is an indisputably vicious procedure. It all too often does not work nor, does it often work well. CPR is, for most patients, extraordinary and may well be futile.[16] The fact is that all of us will experience cardiac arrest at the end of life regardless of our underlying cause of death. For all of us, at some point, CPR will be futile. The decision not to resuscitate should be separate from any other decision regarding withholding or withdrawing other life-sustaining treatments.

If CPR will not permit the patient to leave the hospital, or if the patient refuses it, it should be neither provided nor pushed. Where the decision to place a DNR order in the patient's chart is uncontroversial, the physician need only consult with other physicians or an ethics committee.[17] Physicians are also allowed to stop a futile resuscitation procedure in process.[18] In fact, that is how most patients who are full code die. The resuscitation attempt is finally, after some length of time, deemed to have failed.

Chemical codes—or partial codes that proscribe chest compressions and defibrillation but allow medications—are only generally "doomed from the start."[19] When a patient's heart is stopped she is not breathing. Without chest compressions or defibrillation, the patient has no circulation. Therefore, the medications administered to the patient during CPR just go nowhere; they might as well not be provided. Chemical codes are frankly dishonest; they permit a physician to escape a hard discussion with the patient and her family. The physician's discomfort at discussing a DNR with a patient or the patient's decision-maker is not a reason to write a chemical code order.

The Uniform Health-Care Decisions Act, promulgated by the Uniform Law Commissioners, the American Bar Association, and the American Association of Retired Persons, directs that a health care provider or health care institution may decline to comply with an individual health care instruction or health care decision that requires medically ineffective health care or health care contrary to generally accepted health care standards applicable to the health care provider or institution. The act defines "medically ineffective health care" as treatment offering no benefit.

The act further states:

> A health care provider or health care institution that declines to comply with an individual health care instruction or health care decision shall do all of the following: (a) promptly inform the patient, if possible, and any person then authorized to make health care decisions for the patient; (b) unless the patient or person then authorized to make health care decisions for the patient refuses assistance, then immediately make all reasonable efforts to assist in the transfer of the patient to another health care provider or institution that is willing to comply with the instruction or decision; and (c) provide continuing

care to the patient until a transfer can be accomplished or until it appears that a transfer cannot be accomplished. In all cases, appropriate pain relief and other palliative care shall be continued.[20]

It must be understood–determining that a medical treatment is futile does not mean that we abandon the patient. We *always* care for the patient with compassion. The term *patient* comes from the Latin word *passio*, to suffer, which is also the root of *compassion*. This understanding means that although a treatment may itself be futile, the patient is never futile. *Care and compassion are never futile.*

Many medical treatments may be futile but never so good nursing care. Nursing care is *always* provided. It includes the administration of medications for pain and dyspnea, repositioning to avoid wounds, and keeping the patient clean and as comfortable as possible. Even if a patient dies a few minutes after life-sustaining treatment is withdrawn, comfort measures are always to be compassionately provided.

Conflicts over Futile Treatment

Most conflicts over futile treatment occur when the physician knows that further life-sustaining treatment would be futile and the patient, the patient's decision-maker and/or the patient's family demand it. Much less common are the cases in which a patient or family wishes to withdraw or withhold life-sustaining treatment and the healthcare team wants to continue it. In either case, generally, the family is making decisions for the patient who lacks decision-making capacity.

Conflicts frequently occur when a decision has to be made between giving a mechanically ventilated patient a tracheostomy and withdrawing the ventilator. A patient cannot receive ventilator treatment from a tube down her throat for an extended period without considerable damage. After a period, a tracheostomy must be performed if mechanical ventilation is to be continued. A tracheostomy is a surgical procedure to create an opening through the neck into the trachea. A tube is then placed through this opening to the ventilator. Artificial ventilation is so unpleasant that high doses of sedatives are required so that the patient does not "buck" the ventilator.

In most general cases, the patient has no advance directive or POLST and her preferences regarding life-sustaining treatment are unknown. The physician estimates the patient's best interests from a specific point of view, taking into account the patient's previously expressed values and the appropriateness (or futility) of life-sustaining treatment. The family's perspective and estimation of the patient's best interests is completely different. The family, in hopes of a miraculous cure, demands all possible life-sustaining treatments. This leads to the following scenario: The patient will never leave the intensive care unit. She has no quality of life because she cannot appreciate or experience being alive. The patient is suffering, and she cannot die gently or peacefully without permission. This means that the healthcare team must advocate for the patient's gentle death in the face of fierce and emotional opposition from the family, who insists that the patient's mere biological life must be sustained at all costs, indefinitely.

There are many reasons for a patient or her family, generally adult children, to demand aggressive yet ultimately futile treatment. For example, a child may demand futile treatment for a patient if the child feels guilt for not visiting the patient regularly or for delay in taking the patient to a physician promptly. A child may also demand futile treatment for a patient if the patient had been financially supporting the child or if the child will lose her home upon the death of the patient. Finally, a child may demand futile treatment for even permanently nonresponsive patients if the patient has been an active, life-long substance abuser and the child is searching for reconciliation, regardless of the fact that catharsis will most likely never be realized.

Of course, with regard to treatment, "everything possible" really means "everything reasonable." Absolutely futile treatment is never to be provided. However, even healthcare providers contribute to over-doing "everything possible." We can always do something more or do something longer or try something else. If we continue what we are doing, or if we do everything that we can think of, we think that we might save the patient. Sadly, more often than not a moribund patient permanently dependent on life-sustaining treatment is the result. Recall that the goal of medicine is not only to have a positive effect on the patient's biological life systems but must try to produce an effect that the patient has the capacity to appreciate as a benefit. Although a family's goal may be a miracle, it is not an appropriate medical goal.

It is not effective to repeat to a grieving family that further treatment is futile. The "family that does not get it" is a patronizing phrase to describe relatives who appear to be incapable of understanding the patient's quality of life and prognosis. The most common sources of escalating conflict with such a family are the healthcare team's mislabeling of the conflict, the healthcare team's overemphasis on facts rather than emotions, the family's lack of control, mixed messages to the family from the medical team and, most importantly, the family's mistrust of the healthcare team. For example, the family may decide that the patient is a "fighter," that the present illness is just one more from which the patient will recover, and they want "everything possible" to be done.[21]

Before branding the family as one "who doesn't get it," healthcare providers need to look at much more than just the urgency of the need for a decision—an exceptionally difficult task for the inexperienced. Typically, families who "don't get it" look only at the credibility and trustworthiness of the healthcare team or of the hospital itself. "Just as definitive medical therapy usually requires accurate identification of the disease, so does successful negotiation with families usually depend on identification of the important issues to be negotiated."[22]

(Note that surgeons are privileged in that they make futility decisions by refusing requests to operate on patients that they state are "inoperable.")

Frequently, healthcare providers focus on facts rather than the family's emotions, which range from fear and anger to disappointment, ambivalence, and guilt. Conflicts over futility allow the family to put off the difficult work of grief. The healthcare team usually chooses only to look at the urgency of the decision and decides that the family does not understand the patient's fragile condition. Then the team attempts to bring the family to understanding with "an avalanche of medical explanations."[23]

However, the facts about the patient's condition and treatments may be irrelevant to the family's understanding and decision-making. If we do not acknowledge the emotions with which the family is coping, our repeated recital of the facts, ever louder and more ardent, will not solve the problem. Then, having reinforced our "(mis)impression" that "the family doesn't get it," we make even more efforts to make certain that they understand the facts with another brick wall of information. Thus, the family just becomes all the more intractable, all the more entrenched. Finally, the ethics committee is called in. The hospital's risk manager is generally called as well as the family often threatens to sue for malpractice.

The family's perceived lack of control may also underline a demand for aggressive treatment. The family may be actively chasing the physicians in order to obtain information. This situation inevitably leaves family members feeling that they don't know what's happening and that they have no control over the plan of care for their loved one. Lack of communication and the inability to participate in their loved one's plan of care inevitably results in frustration, anger, and an over-riding emotional need to demonstrate *some* control over the situation, no matter how irrational that control may be. One of the most common ways for the family to "seize control" is to demand futile and aggressive treatment. Requests for futile treatment are often a desperate attempt by the family to assert themselves and regain some sense of determination and authority over the patient's treatment in a situation they do not fully understand.

Mixed messages can also underlie a family's demand for aggressive treatment. Often times, during most patients' stays in an intensive care unit patients and families are pushed information by too many members of the healthcare team, including: clinical social workers, nurses, technicians, residents, attending physicians, and consultants. Most members of the team convey both information and their personal opinions, in individual attempts to advocate for the patient. However, without a lead physician that the family trusts, the family receives too much information—sometimes conflicting—and altogether too many opinions. The family's understanding of the patient's prognosis is likely to depend on who has spoken to them most recently, most persuasively, or with the most positive and emotionally hopeful statements.[24]

Case 9-2. A Daughter's Demand for Aggressive Treatment.

Diane Mason, a seventy-four-year-old woman, has lived alone in her own home for six years following the death of her husband. Her physician first meets her when she is brought to the clinic by her daughter, Jenn. One day, Diane does not answer when Jenn calls to check up on her. Four hours later, Jenn finds Diane passed out on her kitchen floor. At the clinic, the admitting nurse takes Diane's blood pressure; it is very high. Jenn tells Diane's physician that Diane drinks and her drinking has become considerably heavier after the death of her husband. Diane is admitted to the hospital for assessment of her hypertension.

Diane does not want to be in the hospital. She is afraid. Her late husband went to the hospital and he did not come out alive. Jenn, on the other hand, is very concerned about Diane's health. After a careful assessment, Diane is discharged from the hospital with a handful of prescriptions and a warning by her physician that if she does not take the medications, she risks a stroke. He also says that she needs to stop drinking.

Diane is noncompliant. She cancels clinic appointments and does not reschedule them. Jenn becomes even more concerned. She calls Diane's physician to report that Diane refuses to take her medications and her drinking has only become heavier. The physician asks Jenn to drive Diane to the clinic immediately.

Diane's physician takes an hour out of his busy schedule to talk to Diane. He carefully reiterates the risk of a stroke or heart attack. He re-emphasizes the importance of taking the medications and to stop drinking. When her physician asks Diane why she does not take the medications, she says that she does not like doctors or pills and that she came to the clinic only because Jenn forced her. Diane states: "I don't want to die on a machine with tubes everywhere." Diane refuses to fill out an advance directive., saying, "I don't like doctors and I don't want to be here." She storms out the door with Jenn following apologetically.

A few weeks later, Diane tells Jenn early in the morning that she has a bad headache and does not feel well. Jenn cannot leave work to take Diane to the hospital and Diane refuses Jenn's offer to call 911. Jenn arrives at Diane's home six hours later and finds Diane unresponsive on the floor of her kitchen and calls 911.

In the emergency room, Diane is diagnosed with a massive cerebral hemorrhage. She is paralyzed, and her eyes are unresponsive to light. Diane is in a coma. Diane's physician meets with Jenn and explains Diane's condition and poor prognosis. He tells Jenn that, even if Diane survives, she will have massive brain damage.

Jenn wants "everything done," including ventilator support. Jenn tells one of Diane's nurses that she feels guilty for not leaving work and calling 911 when Diane first reported her symptoms. Diane's physician tells Jenn that there was no way to avoid Diane's present condition, and reminds Jenn that Diane does not "want to die on a machine." However, Jenn refuses to agree to limit aggressive treatment.

Discussion Questions

- Should we give Jenn time to grieve before withdrawing aggressive treatment?

- How much time should we give Jenn? How long does it take to grieve a complicated loss?

- If Diane survives, with massive brain damage, do we give her a gastrostomy tube and discharge her to a long-term skilled nursing facility? Or do we place Diane on hospice and let her die naturally?

- Which of these options will help Diane to resolve her grief?

Case 9-3. The Suicide Attempt.

Joseph North, a twenty-year-old man, has a fight with his girlfriend over his cell phone. After she hangs up on him, Joseph reaches below the couch that he is sitting on and pulls out a shotgun. He shakily puts the shotgun in his mouth and pulls the trigger. He does not succeed in killing himself. Joseph succeeds only in shooting off his face and part of his brain. He remains alive. The North family tries to find meaning in this senseless tragedy. They approach the physicians about organ donation. They are ready to let Joseph go. Before removing life-sustaining treatments, the intensivist calls for a neurology consultation.

A neurologist visits Joseph and the North family. The neurologist states that he can put a plate on Joseph's head and, if the operation is successful, may allow him to sit up in a wheelchair. Needless to say, the North family believes him, and the neurologist becomes the family's new best friend. However, a family conference is held by the intensivist and another neurologist who gives the family the most likely facts. The North family decides not to do the surgery. Joseph is not a candidate for organ donation as he is not brain dead and he breathes when ventilator support is stopped for a few minutes. He dies two days later with his entire family and his girlfriend present.

Discussion Questions

- Does the fact that Joseph's situation was caused by attempted suicide mean that he would lack the capacity to make a decision to withdraw life-sustaining treatment?

- Is withdrawal of life-sustaining treatment complicity in Joseph's suicide?

Case 9-4. Xigris.

On January 16, 2011, Howard Crame—a patient from a skilled nursing facility—is admitted to a small community hospital with aspiration pneumonia, respiratory failure, and hypotension. He is eighty-six years old, has end-stage dementia, diabetes, stage four wounds down to the bone, a gastrostomy tube, and chronic congestive heart failure. This is his fourth episode of pneumonia in three months. Howard's family asks for "everything" to be done and specifically mention Xigris, a new drug for the treatment of severe sepsis which was approved by the FDA in 2001. They ask the physicians at the community hospital for the drug, but the pharmacy formulary does not include it. The community hospital is therefore obliged to send the patient to the regional medical center that is able to administer the drug.

On arrival at the regional medical center, Howard is hypotensive, has a high white cell count, a raised temperature, bilateral infiltrates, and Gram-positive bacteria growing from two blood cultures. These are all inclusion criteria for administering Xigris, so Xigris is administered. Two days later, Howard's status is not improving. He requires mechanical ventilation and continuous infusion of a vasopressor to maintain his blood pressure. Howard responds to external pain stimulus by groaning and does not follow commands. Four days after arrival at the regional medical center, Howard dies in the course of a fifty-minute resuscitation attempt. Xigris did not save him.

In October of 2011, Eli Lilly and Company withdrew Xigris from all markets following results of a study that showed that Xigris did not reduce mortality in patients with septic shock in any statistically significant manner. Xigris had cost $8,000 per treatment course. However, given the relative risk of death after treatment with Xigris, "the cost effectiveness of treating patients with an APACHE II score [to predict hospital mortality] of 24 or less increased to $575,054 per life-year gained when the Food and Drug Administration's estimates of effectiveness were considered."[25]

Discussion Questions

- What are the inclusion criteria for administering Xigris? If the patients to whom we administered Xigris were so sick, why should we expect anything, including Xigris, to save them?

- How often do you think that patients in Howard's situation die? How often do they live?

- Why did the FDA overestimate Xigris's effectiveness and then, when it proved ineffective, made Eli Lilly take it off the market?

The Cost of Futile Treatment and the Chronically Critically Ill Patient

Advances in life-sustaining treatment have resulted in more patients surviving acute illness. However, these advances have created a growing population of chronically ill patients. A chronically critically ill patient is defined as a patient who is dependent on life-sustaining treatment for an indeterminate and long-term period of time without reasonable hope of recovery. An intervention's inability to end dependence on life-sustaining treatment is a definition of a futile intervention. Chronically critically ill patients neither die during the acute period of their illnesses nor fully recover no matter what interventions are provided. There are an estimated on 100,000 chronically critically ill patients in the United States and the number is growing. It costs an estimated $20 billion per year to treat these patients, excluding the cost of warehousing them in sub-acute, long-term ventilator facilities, rehabilitation facilities, or skilled nursing facilities which accept ventilator patients to which eighty percent are discharged.[26] Although chronically critically ill patients represent about ten percent of those patients receiving mechanical ventilation, they account for twenty to forty percent of intensive care unit beds and represent about thirteen percent of all hospital costs.[27] Providing mechanical ventilation to chronically ill patients exceeds $200,000 for each quality-adjusted life year gained.[28]

Most chronically critically ill patients experience respiratory failure and are ventilator-dependent. They also experience a myriad of other conditions not the least of which includes prolonged coma or other brain dysfunction. Most are at an increased risk of infection. Patients who can express themselves report pain, dyspnea, depression, and anxiety from the inability to communicate during endotracheal intubation.[29] Nearly all chronically critically ill patients who survive extubation have severe impairments of cognition and physical function.[30] Most are warehoused in skilled nursing, inpatient rehabilitation, and chronic ventilator facilities.[31] Patient stays in these facilities are expensive and few families can afford them for long. Most of the stays are funded by the taxpayers.

We have to wonder whether prolonged mechanical ventilation with no hope of independent living due to cognitive and physical dysfunctions, is worthwhile to the truncated quality of life of these patients. The question is how long we can afford to warehouse long-term ventilator patients and other chronically critically ill patients.

Chapter 10. Healthcare Allocation

Throughout the United States medical treatment is influenced by two driving forces. The first is the technological imperative: if we have the technology, we use it. The second is the treatment imperative: if we have the treatment, we use it. What this means is that healthcare costs are driven by supply, not demand. However, eventually demand always catches up with supply. The summation of this scenario is that we simply do not seem to know when enough is enough.

Healthcare spending in the United States in 2014 was 17.1 percent of Gross Domestic Product (GDP). This is compared to about 5.0 percent in 1960.[1] The drivers of the increase include the development of new, expensive drugs of uncertain benefit and an increase in direct-to-consumer advertising contributing to the greater use of prescription drugs.[2] Over the next decade, healthcare expenditures will account for 20 percent of the United States Gross Domestic Product. Healthcare spending growth in the United States for 2015–25 is projected to average 5.8 percent— 1.3 percentage points faster than growth in the GDP—and to represent 20.1 percent of the total economy by 2025.[3] The obvious question is how much we can be spending on healthcare going forward.

The regional supply of health care resources (such as hospital beds, intensive care unit beds, and imaging equipment) is the driver of the intensity of care, *not the patient's condition*.[4] If a medical center has three Computerized Tomography (CT) scan machines, all three will be in constant use whether scans are needed or not. The more CT scanners are available, the more CT scans patients will receive, yet the actual problem is not technology or treatment. The real problem is how we utilize technology and proceed with pushing treatment.

We must admit that futile life-sustaining treatment can lead only to dying patients with miserable outcomes and miserable deaths. "Our doctors are equally subject to technology's allure. They learn in medical school to assess, treat, and cure. They then move into a hospital culture where a death, even among the aged, is seen as a failure."[5]

The data released on the Dartmouth Atlas website (www.dartmouthatlas.org) illustrates the problems of the technological and treatment imperatives. Medicare data was analyzed after controlling for patient age, gender, race, tumor type, and non-cancer chronic conditions. The Dartmouth data shows that the chances that a patient with advanced cancer will die in the hospital in 2010 varied from thirteen percent to 150 percent and the days spent in intensive care units (ICUs) in the last month of life varied by five hundred percent. The differences depended on the medical center providing the treatment and included National Cancer Institute-designated Cancer Centers.

The Dartmouth data also shows that Medicare patients in higher-spending regions receive more treatment due to oversupply of medical resources. Higher-spending regions have more hospital beds, more intensive care unit beds, more physicians, and more specialists. Patients in high-spending regions are hospitalized more frequently, spend more time in the ICU, see more physicians more frequently, and receive more diagnostic tests than identical patients in lower-spending regions. In regions where there are more hospital beds, more patients are admitted to the hospital and Medicare spends more on hospital care. In regions where there are more intensive care unit beds, more patients are treated in the ICU and Medicare spends more on ICU care. In regions where more CT scanners are available, patients will receive more CT scans and Medicare will pay accordingly.

The strange fact is that there are extreme differences in the treatment of cancer patients throughout the United States. For example, according to the Dartmouth data, inpatient spending per decedent in the last six months of life varied from $9,636 in Utah to $24,099 in New York. Even if the cost of a single treatment, such as a CT scan, were the same across all states, these differences demonstrate that considerably more treatment is given in New York than in Utah. Obviously, treatment decisions are not always matched to patient conditions. Otherwise, why would dying patients in one region receive more futile treatment than dying patients in another region? Why would dying patients in one medical center receive more futile treatment than in other medical centers?[6] Decisions to provide futile treatment are impacted by the regions and institutions providing it.

We must recognize that there is a fundamental disconnect between what dying cancer patients want in their last days and the treatment imperative that drives physicians. "Most patients with cancer who are approaching the end of their lives prefer supportive care that minimizes symptoms and their days in the hospital. Unfortunately, the care patients receive does not always reflect their own preferences, but rather the prevailing styles of treatment in the regions and health care systems where they happen to receive cancer treatment."[7]

Many studies analyzing Medicare data have determined that higher spending does not result in better quality of care. For example, regions experiencing the greatest increase in health care spending for heart attack patients did not exhibit rapid improvements in health outcomes.[8]

The share of Medicare payments going to patients in their last year of life is about twenty-seven percent of the total Medicare budget.[9] Medicare is estimated to be $660 billion in debt by 2023. Reducing annual growth in per capita spending from the national average of 3.5 percent to 2.4 percent by using hospice and other palliative care management would leave Medicare with a surplus of $758 billion, *a cumulative savings of $1.42 trillion.*[10]

Despite these numbers, it appears that the "full court press" approach and aggressive treatment is often the easiest route; no difficult conversations need to take place and no hard decisions need to be made. However, the Medicare data regarding health outcomes shows that limiting end-of-life treatment is far less about rationing and more about "good medicine." "Few of us want to die in an intensive care unit strapped to a bed under fluorescent lights separated from our loved ones."[11]

We can work to rectify poor end-of-life treatment if physicians, patients, and families receive quality education about end-of-life issues. We can help to rectify poor end-of-life treatment if we are careful to achieve acceptable informed choice, advance directives, and POLST. Conversations between patients and physicians, and patients and their families, can result in better, compassionate end-of-life treatment. Perhaps what is needed most is public service education about end-of-life issues.

It may be that some expensive, rarely successful aggressive treatments might be appropriate. However, cost must be a factor. Recalling Schneiderman: we do not treat one hundred patients in the hope of achieving one successful outlier. Dying patients do not have an unqualified right to expensive treatment of uncertain value. No patient has the right to have his life prolonged with aggressive and expensive treatment at a huge and disproportionate cost with unlikely outcome.

Good palliative care not only results in good deaths, it drives end-of-life treatment costs down. With appropriate education about good end-of-life practices and appropriate conversations between physicians and patients, patients' informed choices will result in less expense and better quality of life at the end.

Some argue that rationing health care will lead to euthanasia as a way to control costs. To the contrary, it is far more likely that massive overspending and massive over-treatment will lead to euthanasia. However, making an appropriate decision to let biological life go is not euthanasia. It is allowing a patient to die—a decision fundamentally rooted in human compassion. Both the intention of the agent and the actions leading up to the death are completely different. If we make appropriate decisions about life-sustaining treatment and provide better end-of-life treatment, then we will not be driven toward euthanasia as a way to control costs and ensure better quality of life. Why not do everything that *should* be done and not everything that *can* be done?

Chapter 11. Ethics Committees

Case 11-1. A Homeless Man.

A homeless man is found unconscious on the street. He is brought by the paramedics to the emergency department of a major medical center as a John Doe. He is fingerprinted by the local police department but has no criminal record–they cannot determine his identity. The medical center social worker reaches out to the local homeless shelters but no one can identify John Doe. Therefore, John Doe has no one to make decisions for him and no identity. John Doe is found to have a bleed in his brainstem. He has no respiratory drive and is on a ventilator. The neurosurgeons deem John Doe an inoperable case.

After five days, John Doe is given a tracheostomy for long-term ventilator support. John Doe cannot be weaned from the ventilator. He remains a full code. John Doe's nurses contact the ethics committee and the medical center's ethicist becomes involved.

The ethicist reviews the chart and the ethical values involved. There are three questions that came to primacy. The first is whether John Doe should have a Do-Not-Resuscitate order. The second question is whether John Doe should be given a gastrostomy tube for artificial nutrition. The third question is whether John Doe's ventilator should be withdrawn, and John Doe be allowed to die or, alternatively, whether John Doe should remain on the ventilator, be given a gastrostomy tube, and sent to a facility that accepts long-term ventilator patients.

The ethicist calls for a surrogate committee to make decisions for John Doe. The surrogate committee is comprised of the head of the ethics committee, a physician, one of John Doe's nurses, the intensivist caring for John Doe, a chaplain, a social worker, and a member of the local community. The surrogate committee meets by conference call.

The ethicist presents the case with the questions, along with her recommendation. The surrogate committee members discuss John Doe's quality of life. They determine, because John Doe will never regain consciousness, that John Doe has no quality of life. The committee also determines that further life-sustaining treatment would be futile because John Doe will never be able to appreciate its benefits. The surrogate committee recommends that the intensivist write a DNR, that John Doe's ventilator be withdrawn, and comfort care provided.

Discussion Questions

- Do you believe that the surrogate committee included all persons who should participate in decision-making for John Doe?

- Do you believe that the intensivist can write a DNR order without getting John Doe's consent, or that he should remain full code?

- Do you believe that the surrogate committee had the right to allow John Doe to die or should he have been given a tracheostomy and gastrostomy tube and sent to a facility that accepts long-term ventilator patients?

An ethics committee is an entity within a medical center but separate from it. An ethics committee is typically comprised of: a physician chairperson, an ethics consultant with a graduate degree in bioethics, a director of nursing, a medical social worker, and a chaplain. An ethics committee also includes a member of the community at large whose ethnicity and culture reflect the demographic of the patients that are admitted to the medical center. Neither a risk manager nor a utilization planner should be on an ethics committee as the goal of the committee is to make decisions and approve policies as a separate entity from the medical center—fully outside of financial considerations. The ethics committee assures that decisions and recommendations are informed solely by ethical principles.

A medical center must have a futility policy if the medical center is to function. The best futility policies set forth a definition of futile treatment as well as a process by which disputes can be resolved. Processes without definitions lead to circular discussions that in turn lead nowhere fast. Definitions without processes mean that physicians can make unilateral decisions without allowing anyone else to be heard. Most medical center policies describe the conditions of limiting an obligation to provide futile treatment and provide a mechanism for addressing disputes over what physicians conclude are futile treatments. Almost all futility policies state that physicians are not obligated to continue life-sustaining treatment for patients who have been determined to be permanently unconscious or who are permanently dependent on the intensive care unit for survival.

Medical center futility policies must recognize the vulnerability of patients and their surrogates (or family members) in futility determinations. They must address the differential in power between the health care professionals, the institution, and the patients, surrogates, and/or families in making a futility determination. *They must also recognize that palliative care is never futile and must always be provided.*

Medical center futility policies must also caution against healthcare providers making quality-of-life determinations for patients receiving futile treatment. Quality-of-life judgments are made from the perspective of patients with the essential input of medical expertise by the treating physicians. Physicians and other healthcare professionals should not make quality-of-life judgments for patients independently of patients' expressed values. This is equally applicable to surrogate decision-makers and/or patients' families.

In a futility policy the primary, treating, or designated physician is responsible for determining whether a treatment or medical intervention is medically ineffective. The physician *and* the patient (or the patient's decision-maker) determine whether a treatment is ultimately beneficial or burdensome.

The physician carefully and thoroughly explains to the patient, the patient's decision-maker, and/or the patient's family, the nature of the patient's condition, his or her prognosis, and what comfort-care treatments will be provided—namely palliative care. The physician must always explain the rationale and basis for the determination that further aggressive treatment is futile. This methodology reflects the informed choice process.

If the patient, the patient's decision-maker, and/or the patient's family do not accept the judgement of the physician, the following may occur:

- The primary physician provides the patient, the patient's decision-maker, and/or the patient's family with a reasonable and agreed-upon period—of no more than seven days—to obtain another medical evaluation of the treatment. The physician may provide the names of other qualified physicians who can give an independent second opinion.

- A family conference is held with a physician and the ethics consultant and may include others, such as a medical social worker and a chaplain. In the past, family conferences have proven to be an effective way to inform the patient, the patient's decision-maker, and/or the patient's family of the determination that a treatment or intervention is futile. Ideally, the policy will require that a family conference be held within forty-eight hours of the patient's admission to the intensive care unit.

If a resolution can be reached, in which all agree that the treatment is futile, the treatment is withheld or withdrawn. However, if a resolution cannot be reached, the physician may arrange for a transfer to another facility and continue the existing treatments for a trial period of not more than seven days. After seven days, the physician will reassess the patient's condition and the appropriate treatments with the patient, the patient's decision-maker, and/or the patient's family. If a resolution still cannot be reached and the transfer of the patient is virtually impossible, and the treatment provided during the trial period continues to be futile, then the treatment may be unilaterally withheld or withdrawn. For example, the treating physician may write a Do-Not-Resuscitate (DNR) order.

An ethics consultation referral may be initiated by anyone, including:

- A patient
- A patient's surrogate decision-maker or agent under an advance directive
- A physician
- Any clinician treating the patient, including: certified nursing assistants, nurses, respiratory therapists, physical therapists, occupational therapists, dietitians, social workers, and chaplains
- Any associate of the medical center, including housekeeping or environmental services personnel

A physician's order should never be necessary to initiate an ethics consultation and the policy must allow for referrals to be made anonymously. Moreover, ethics determinations are recommendations, not directives.

In most medical centers, certain treatments or intervals trigger an automatic ethics consultation, including, but not limited to:

- Intensive care unit stay greater than seven days
- Ventilator dependence for more than six days
- Profound neurologic deficit
- Multiple decubitus ulcers
- Multi-system failure or multi-organ failure
- Recurrent aspiration pneumonia complicating existing conditions
- Multiple re-admissions to the hospital
- Pain and other end-of-life symptoms not being adequately addressed
- Profound paralysis following a post-cerebrovascular accident (CVA)
- End-stage dementia
- Patient noncompliance
- A chemical code order in place
- Any other significant clinical criteria that poses an ethical issue

Ethics consultations need to be more than discussion, facilitation, and mediation. Once a dispute about futile treatment takes place between a treating physician and a patient—the patient's decision-maker and/or the patient's family—and multiple conferences have failed, we find we need much more than process. Some ethics consultants believe that their only role in such a dispute is to let all parties be heard and then mediate between them. Unfortunately, processes without definitions tend to lead nowhere.

In mediation, the ethics consultant:

- Convenes the entire interdisciplinary medical team
- Encourages the interdisciplinary team's transparency
- Frames, reframes, and restates everything said in the meeting until all participants understand the positions of the interdisciplinary team and the patient or patient's decision-maker
- Offer options such as time-limited trials of treatment after which the patient's medical condition is re-assessed
- Supports the patient or decision-maker
- Supports the interdisciplinary medical team

Clinical ethics mediation is most effectively accomplished face-to-face but sometimes surrogate decision-makers make themselves scarce. Skype or another interactive video system may be used to involve an otherwise unavailable surrogate.

Note, however, that limiting the ethics consultant to a mediator role disempowers the interdisciplinary team's ability to treat the patient appropriately. Usually, the surrogate's decision overrides that of the interdisciplinary team or the case ends up in court. The futility policy must contain a definition of futile treatment that will limit end-of-life treatment with patients who have no quality of life and who are only suffering in "suspended animation."

If no agreement can be made between the physicians and the patient (or the patient's decision-maker) and there is no definition of futility in the medical center's futility policy, then one of two other approaches may be taken. The first approach is easy, eliminates conflict, and is completely unethical. Under the unethical approach—say, with a patient on a ventilator who has no quality of life—we would give the patient a gastrostomy tube, a tracheostomy for mechanical ventilation, a DNR, and then "turf" the patient to an outside sub-acute facility that takes permanent ventilator patients. This is unethical because we are allowing the patient to suffer for the sake of expediency. We should not make a patient with futile treatment some other institution's problem, especially where the futile treatment will probably continue to be provided.

The better approach, when conflict between a patient, a patient's decision-maker and/or the patient's family cannot be resolved, allows the physicians to write orders that are consistent with the patient's best interests. Under this approach, life-sustaining treatment may be withheld or withdrawn by the physician unilaterally. Three to five days should be given prior to executing the orders to enable the family to find another facility or physician who will provide the futile treatment. Palliative care is always appropriate. Ethics consultants attempt to set limits on futile treatment as well as to respond to medical center (and social) concerns about resources.

A surrogate decision-making committee is a subcommittee of an ethics committee. Surrogate decision-making policies provide a process for committee members to make medical treatment decisions on behalf of an adult patient who lacks even an unconventional surrogate decision-maker. These patients are unrepresented or "unbefriended." Surrogate committees came into being because of the difficulty, time, and expense of a medical center asking a probate court judge to rule that an employee of the medical center be named as conservator. A conservator is authorized to make medical decisions for a patient. The probate judge may of course prefer to order a public conservator to represent the patient. This can, however, become a nightmare for all parties, as most public conservators know nothing about futile treatment but do know how to preserve a biological life.

Decisions made without clear knowledge of an unrepresented patient's specific treatment preferences must be in the patient's best interest, taking into consideration the patient's personal history, values, and beliefs to the extent that these are known. Decisions about treatment must be made with a focus on the patient's interests and not the interests of providers, the institution, or other affected parties. Appropriate healthcare decisions include both the provision of needed medical treatment and the avoidance of futile treatment.

Surrogate committee policies are largely procedural in nature and are intended to support the medical center's informed choice policy.

A surrogate decision-making committee should be comprised of all of the following:

- A physician member of the ethics committee
- An attending physician
- A nurse familiar with the patient
- A chaplain
- A medical social worker familiar with the patient
- An ethics consultant
- A person who does not provide direct patient care

- A community member at large

A surrogate may not make a medical treatment decision that is biased as to the patient's age, sexual orientation, gender, gender identity, gender expression, race, color, religion, ancestry, national origin, disability, or marital status. *The patient's ability to pay for health care services is ethically irrelevant, although concerns about distributive justice may be considered.*

In order to determine the appropriate medical treatment for the patient, the surrogate committee should review the diagnosis and prognosis of the patient and then determine the appropriate goals of care by weighing the following considerations:

- The patient's previously expressed wishes if any and to the extent known
- Relief of suffering and pain
- Improvement of medical condition
- Recovery of cognitive functions
- Quality and extent of life sustained
- Degree of intrusiveness
- The risk and discomfort of treatment

The purpose of ethics rounds is to discuss difficult cases proactively before futility disputes occur. The ethics consultant assists participants by clarifying concepts and offering possible solutions to problems, as well as educating the participants about ethical principles. The ethics consultant should also provide support to participants as they work in ethically significant cases.

Chapter 12. Palliative Sedation

Case 12-1. Palliative Sedation and Quality of Life.

Jaspar Shannon is fifty-four years old and has amyotrophic lateral sclerosis, also known as ALS or Lou Gehrig's disease. Over the last few months, Jaspar has become more and more dependent on his mother, Joan, who is his caregiver. Jaspar is bedbound, is having great difficulty swallowing, and is beginning to have trouble breathing. Jaspar has refused life-sustaining treatments such as artificial nutrition and hydration and mechanical ventilation. Physician-assisted suicide is unavailable in his state. However, even if it were legal, Jaspar could not swallow the pills.

Jaspar is depressed and frightened about his rapid decline. He frequently states, to the sorrow of his mother: "I need this to be over. I can't take any more." He asks his mother and his nurses to kill him to put him out of his misery. They refuse, some out of legal and professional repercussions, others from heartbreak.

Discussion Questions

- What is Jasper's emotional and spiritual state? What can we do to help him? Do you believe that Jaspar is asking to die because he is depressed? Or is there another reason?

- If Jaspar does not have access to physician-assisted suicide, or because his swallowing is impaired and he cannot take the pills, what do we do to make his quality of life better?

When a patient is given the usual doses of medication, yet is still suffering, we have recourse to several "last resort" options, such as:

- Palliative sedation
- Voluntarily stopping eating and drinking
- The principle of double effect
- Physician-assisted suicide
- Voluntary euthanasia
- Nonvoluntary euthanasia
- Involuntary euthanasia

Unrelieved pain and other end-of-life symptoms are dehumanizing. When we fail to ease suffering appropriately, we are treating the patient as an animal. Moreover, a patient cannot die with unrelieved symptoms. Dying at this stage is a matter of relaxation and surrender, a matter of saying "Yes" to the end, of welcoming death as the comfort of an old friend. A suffering patient cannot relax enough to let his or her biological life go. A last resort option, palliative sedation, may be necessary. Palliative sedation is the deliberate lowering of consciousness, with sedatives, so that the patient is no longer suffering. Palliative sedation is commonly viewed as at the outer edge of the continuum of symptom management, short of death.

In palliative sedation, we increase the level of sedating medications and unconsciousness until the patient's suffering is tolerable. Sedation should be maintained at that level. Once sufficiently sedated the patients' symptoms, burdens, and level of suffering should be regularly assessed. The level of sedation must be adjusted to ensure that the level of suffering is tolerable.

Palliative sedation is used for terminally ill patients with unrelieved symptoms, burn patients, trauma patients, and in the intensive care unit so that patients can tolerate mechanical ventilation. This chapter will concentrate on the use of palliative sedation at the end of life. When palliative sedation is the appropriate treatment for a terminally ill patient, all other life-sustaining treatments have been withheld or withdrawn, including: antibiotics, mechanical ventilation, artificial nutrition, and hydration. At this point, such measures will only prolong the patient's dying process without promoting the patient's quality of life.

The term *terminal sedation* incorrectly implies that the sedating medications are the cause of death. The purpose of palliative sedation is to decrease consciousness to relieve suffering or allow treatment, not to cause or hasten death. The level of sedating medication provided is not sufficient to kill the patient under the principle of double effect, discussed in a later chapter. Therefore, the term terminal sedation is inappropriate.

The goal of palliative sedation is the relief of intolerable and intractable suffering. For some patients, total unconsciousness may be necessary. For others, some consciousness may be appropriate so that the patient may be aroused.[1]

Palliative sedation is not euthanasia. Properly administered, the sedatives used in palliative sedation do not hasten or in any way cause death. If palliative sedation were unavailable, suicide and euthanasia would be the inevitable result. Suffering patients would plead with their physicians and families for assisted suicide or voluntary euthanasia as a means of relieving their suffering. Without palliative sedation, we would be forced to resort to mercy-killing patients in order to relieve their suffering. Under these circumstances, gently allowing the patient to die would give way to active euthanasia.

When a patient expresses fear about dying a "bad death" from unrelieved suffering, it is appropriate to inform that patient of the availability of palliative sedation. This is important in regions where physician-assisted suicide is illegal, not practiced, or is otherwise unavailable. Some patients may believe that death during sedation is undignified, but many others will be greatly relieved by the option. For terminally ill patients, palliative sedation is an intervention of last resort to relieve intolerable, intractable suffering.

"Although rendering a patient unconscious to escape suffering is an extraordinary measure, withholding such treatment in certain circumstances would be inhumane."[2] The American Medical Association states that physicians have an ethical obligation to provide palliative sedation for intractable symptoms. "The duty to relieve pain and suffering is central to the physician's role as healer and is an obligation physicians have to their patients."

> It is an accepted and appropriate component of end-of-life care under specific, relatively rare circumstances. When symptoms cannot be diminished through all other means of palliation, including symptom-specific treatments, it is the ethical obligation of a physician to offer palliative sedation to unconsciousness as an option for the relief of intractable symptoms.[3]

The intent in palliative sedation is to relieve the patient's awareness of suffering that is both intolerable and intractable. In this case, the induction and maintenance of a state of unconsciousness may be the only remaining option short of mercy-killing the patient. Palliative sedation in the imminently dying is intended to produce a level of unconsciousness that is sufficient to relieve suffering without hastening death.

There are two types of suffering to think about when considering palliative sedation. The first type is *intolerable suffering*, in which the patient determines what level of suffering he or she can tolerate. Just as the patient's pain is what the patient says it is, suffering is intolerable when the patient says it is. We evaluate whether intolerable suffering is relieved when the level of suffering becomes bearable, always as defined by the patient.

The second type of suffering is *intractable suffering*. Intractable suffering is, as it sounds, suffering that is utterly intolerable and beyond the hope of control, and all other treatments have been tried and failed. Because palliative sedation is an intervention of last resort, it should be offered only when suffering is intractable as well as intolerable and refusing to sedate the patient while trying other treatments would harm the patient.[4] Of course, intractable symptoms may include more than pure pain. Palliative sedation is also available for the following, to name just a few:

- Bleeding
- Delirium
- Dyspnea (shortness of breath)
- Pain
- Seizures
- Deep, open tissue wounds
- Vomiting

Up to thirty-five percent of hospice patients describe their pain as "severe" in the last week of life and twenty-five percent describe their shortness of breath as "unbearable."[5] A patient with chronic obstructive pulmonary disease (COPD) may say to his medical team: "I know how I am going to die. I am going to die gasping for breath." The promise of palliative sedation gives these patients hope for a good death.

The intent of comfort medications is to reduce symptoms without necessarily causing sedation. Palliative sedation is different from the sedation caused by the usual comfort medications. The intent of palliative sedation is to reduce the patient's symptom-burden by deliberately reducing consciousness.

Because of the danger of disguised pain in patients receiving palliative sedation, normal opioids or other pain management agents are continued. Sedation is insufficient if the patient is moaning or grimacing with routine repositioning. Normal pain medication is continued to avoid the possibility of unobservable pain.

Palliative sedation is usually accomplished with benzodiazepines, anesthetics such as Propofol, and both short- and long-acting barbiturates.[6] Because a patient receiving palliative sedation may take up to a week or more to die, many patients may prefer physician-assisted suicide when it is available.

The patient's underlying fatal pathology is the legal and ethical cause of death when we withhold or withdraw life-sustaining treatment. The legal and ethical cause of death also comes down to the fatal pathology if the patient dies while receiving sedation— providing that appropriate non-lethal doses of medication were used.

The intent behind palliative sedation is to relieve suffering without reducing life expectancy. Properly administered, palliative sedation does not involve the administration of a lethal agent. Properly administered, the levels of sedating medications needed to eliminate intolerable and intractable symptoms do not cause death. There also appears to be no difference in time of death between patients who receive palliative sedation at the end of life and those who do not.[7]

The goal or outcome of palliative sedation is relief of suffering. The means by which this goal is pursued is the lowering of consciousness. Palliative sedation, therefore, does not target the causes of suffering. Rather, it lowers a patient's awareness of his or her suffering by reducing consciousness. Palliative sedation should be used only to the degree that it controls symptoms to a level that is tolerable to the patient. Sedated patients may be reassessed continually, and consideration should be given to reversing the sedation if there is reason to believe that the symptom burden has changed and the patient's symptoms will be within tolerable levels.

Palliative sedation is, all told, completely different from physician-assisted suicide and euthanasia. The intent of physician-assisted suicide or euthanasia is to end the patient's suffering by ending the patient's life. In euthanasia and physician-assisted suicide, relief or prevention of suffering is accomplished by facilitating death for the patient who is only suffering and has no hope of getting better. In palliative sedation, death is not used as a means to achieve symptom relief. Rather, death occurs at some point due to the patient's underlying fatal pathology after her suffering is relieved. Palliative sedation is also reversible, unlike physician-assisted suicide and euthanasia.

When a patient expresses fear about dying a "bad death" from unrelieved suffering, it is appropriate to inform that patient of the availability of palliative sedation in areas where physician-assisted suicide is illegal, not practiced, or unavailable. Most patients will express relief with the availability of a "back-up plan" other than hoarding pain medication in case it all becomes too much. As a last resort option, palliative sedation is an alternative to physician-assisted suicide where the physician, the patient, or his or her family or friends have qualms about physician-assisted suicide. On the other hand, many argue that physician-assisted suicide is the option that truly reflects many patients' needs and that it should be provided in accordance with those needs.[8]

It is also appropriate to point out here that the decision for voluntarily stopping eating and drinking (as described below) requires that the patient has full capacity; alternatively, a surrogate decision-maker may use *informed choice* to consent to palliative sedation on behalf of a patient who lacks the necessary decision-making capacity. Consent for palliative sedation may also be made for unbefriended patients without surrogates by an ethics surrogate subcommittee operating under an appropriate policy for palliative sedation.

Separate decisions should be made about utilizing palliative sedation from decisions about artificial nutrition and hydration. Patients who are imminently dying have naturally decreased intake of food and fluids. For a dying patient, artificial nutrition and/or hydration are at high risk of fluid overload, causing congestion, edema, and ascites. Artificial nutrition and hydration is not provided during palliative sedation because it may increase symptoms or may, although rarely, prolong death.

Palliative sedation may also be appropriate for patients who are not imminently dying. The National Hospice and Palliative Care Organization (NHPCO) defines *imminent death* as a prognosis of death within fourteen days. For patients who are not imminently dying, it is important to separate the decision about the appropriateness of artificial nutrition and hydration from the decision about palliative sedation. Each decision should always be based on its own merits. The decision to initiate or continue artificial nutrition and hydration should be based on its relative benefits, burdens, and the patient's quality of life. The decision to use palliative sedation should be based on the need to provide appropriate symptom management to a patient with intolerable, intractable, and unrelieved symptoms.

The concern in using palliative sedation in patients who are not imminently dying and are not receiving artificial nutrition and hydration is that sedation will prevent them from ingesting food and fluids. There is concern, then, that the palliative sedation may contribute to the death. However, artificial nutrition and hydration may be withheld from a patient just as any other life-sustaining treatment may be withheld or withdrawn. If a patient who is not imminently dying dies under palliative sedation, then the legal and ethical cause of death is the patient's fatal pathology.

The use of palliative sedation for existential suffering (such as immense feelings of fear, guilt, and/or shame) reflects the understanding that real suffering can occur even when physical symptoms are well controlled. "Suffering is a more expansive concept than pain. It goes beyond unpleasant sensations or distressing symptoms to encompass the anguish, terror, and hopelessness that dying patients may experience. A dying person who experiences few if any physical symptoms may suffer greatly if he or she feels that life has lost any meaning."[9]

Existential suffering arises from "a loss or interruption of meaning, purpose, or hope in life."[10] Existential suffering may be every shred as intractable as unrelieved physical symptoms. *Attempts to eliminate existential suffering must be taken as seriously as attempts to eliminate physical symptoms.* Existential suffering needs to be addressed by the entire interdisciplinary team, including physicians, nurses, medical social workers, and chaplains. "Whether palliative sedation should be a part of that response is an important, growing, and unresolved question."[11] Unfortunately, the National Hospice and Palliative Care Organization has reserved judgment on the use of palliative sedation for existential symptoms.

In exploring further options, *respite sedation* may be used rather than palliative sedation. Respite sedation is temporary and time-limited, and is utilized to lower consciousness for a period, after which the patient is roused so his symptom-burden can be reassessed to determine if future sedation is appropriate.

Finally, studies show that patients receiving palliative sedation actually live longer than patients with unrelieved symptom-burdens. Those patients receiving palliative sedation lived an average of twelve days versus nine days, compared to patients with unrelieved symptoms.[12]

Case 12-2. Dying at Home.

James Martin is a seventy-three-year-old man with metastatic prostate cancer. He lives with his wife of the same age and his adult children assist with his daily care. When he received his terminal diagnosis, James told his family that he wants to die at home.

James has metastasis to his bones and he has had multiple pathological fractures. He has received palliative radiation. He is bed-bound to decrease the risk of further injury. He is able to take only a few small sips of Pepsi on a sponge, his favorite drink.

James' pain has increased. The doses of opioids prescribed are inadequate and make him unarousable, to the consternation of his family. When he is awake, he cries out in pain. When he is asleep, he moans. James is obviously in constant pain and his family does not know what to do. James is on hospice yet nothing that the hospice team tries works.

The hospice nurse informs James' family about the availability of palliative sedation. However, James would have to be transferred to the hospice inpatient unit to receive palliative sedation. His family does not know what to do.

Discussion Questions

- Is palliative sedation appropriate for James? What about the fact that his family wants him to be responsive?

- James wants to die at home. Is it acceptable to move him so that he can get more intensive treatment?

Case 12-3. Intolerable to the patient or to the family?

Stacy Hall is seventy years old. She has lung cancer due to a long history of smoking. When diagnosed with chronic obstructive pulmonary disease (COPD), she quit smoking and now uses oxygen around the clock. She also uses a benzodiazepine and an opioid, both liquid and long-acting, to control her dyspnea. Her son, Mark, is her primary caregiver although home nurses do visit. Stacy is a sweet and generous woman and is beloved by many friends, neighbors, and her church family. She always has a good word for everyone. Despite her failing health, Stacy shows concerns for others who are struggling.

Stacy sleeps during the day and is awake at night. As a result, Mark is constantly losing sleep. He has a baby monitor next to his bed so that he can hear when his mother needs something.

One night, Stacy becomes confused and agitated. She removes her clothes and her diaper and struggles to get out of her hospital bed in the living room. She refuses her opioids and the benzodiazepines appear to increase, rather than decrease, her agitation. Despite Mark's attention, Stacy falls out of bed onto her shoulder and receives a large slash in her skin.

Mark calls the nursing agency at four in the morning after Stacy falls out of bed. A nurse arrives and tries to assist Mark in getting Stacy in her recliner, but she is so confused, uncooperative, and combative that they nearly drop her. Throughout this, Stacy is gasping for breath. She calls out but neither Mark nor the nurse understand what she is saying. Mark tries to give Stacy more medication, but it does not appear to help Stacy's agitation. Mark is at his wit's end. He is very distressed that Stacy is so agitated and is acting so uncharacteristically. He feels that he cannot tolerate Stacy's agitation one more minute.

Mark learned about palliative sedation on the radio several years ago. He requests palliative sedation for Stacy.

Discussion Questions

- What techniques could Mark and the nurse use to calm Stacy down?
- Would we be sedating Stacy for herself or for Mark?
- Is palliative sedation appropriate for agitation instead of pain?
- Will palliative sedation hasten Stacy's death?

Case 12-4. The Torture Survivor.

Hans is Dutch-Indonesian. He was imprisoned in Indonesia in a concentration camp during World War II. He was twelve years old when he entered the camp. During his imprisonment he saw his friends beheaded right next to him and received beatings that left him near-dead.

Now, Hans is fragile physically and emotionally. He is suffering from end-stage dementia and is always confused. He lives in a residential home for the elderly. His wife, who was also imprisoned in a concentration camp, is too frail to visit Hans.

Every night, Hans experiences night terrors and believes that he is back in the concentration camp. He is frightened, agitated, and always afraid. The staff at the residential home cannot calm him and doses of anti-psychotics and anti-anxiety medication only appear to terrorize him further. As he becomes more frail, his night terrors get worse and now Hans is experiencing flash-backs almost continuously all day.

Discussion Questions

- Is palliative sedation appropriate for Jan's out-of-control symptoms?

- Does it matter that he is still taking sips of water but is refusing food?

- Is there any alternative to make Jan's last days more comfortable short of palliative sedation?

Chapter 13. Voluntarily Stopping Eating and Drinking (VSED)

Case 13-1. Amyotrophic Lateral Sclerosis and Voluntarily Stopping Eating and Drinking.

Larry Shannon is fifty-four years old and has amyotrophic lateral sclerosis, also known as ALS or Lou Gehrig's disease. When he was healthy, he was active and rode his bicycle twenty miles or more a day. Now, Larry is bed-bound. His activities are limited to lying in bed with the television on.

Larry also feels he has become a burden to family and friends. Larry has refused artificial nutrition and hydration or a ventilator and his symptoms continue to worsen. He feels that he is dying too slowly so he asks his physician and nurses for hastened death. As Larry lives in a state where physician-assisted suicide is illegal, he decides to voluntarily stop eating and drinking.

Larry's physician affirms that he has the capacity to make this decision and that the decision makes sense for the patient given his meager quality of life. Larry is already having difficulty swallowing food and fluids. Stopping eating and drinking seems to be the logical next step.

Larry is admitted to home hospice. The hospice nurses and medical director manage Larry's confusion and agitation along the way to his easy and gentle death.

Discussion Questions

- Is it right to assist Larry in dying of dehydration and starvation?

- **Does Larry have capacity to make the choice to stop taking food and liquids? Should he receive a gastrostomy tube regardless of his wishes?**

- **What support do we need to give Larry as he dies?**

Voluntarily stopping eating and drinking (VSED) is another last resort for patients facing the end of life who are not experiencing a quality of life that they wish to tolerate. In VSED, a patient with decision-making capacity refuses food and fluids with the intention of hastening his death. VSED is different from the natural loss of interest in food and fluids experienced by many patients at the end of life.[13]

A patient making an informed choice for VSED has or will refuse all other life-sustaining treatments. Artificial nutrition, hydration, and antibiotics (as well as any other life-sustaining treatments) are withheld or withdrawn prior to VSED since they will only prolong the dying process without promoting the patient's quality of life.

VSED is appropriate when a patient is experiencing intolerable and intractable suffering and is living with a quality of life that is unacceptable to him or her. Quill and Byock point out that reasons why patients choose VSED include: "extreme fatigue, weakness, or debility". Good palliative care should always be provided to patients who opt for VSED.

Some bioethicists view VSED as a form of suicide. However, VSED is fundamentally a decision to forego life-sustaining treatment. A patient with decision-making capacity has a virtually absolute right to refuse any and all life-sustaining treatment, even at the cost of death.[14] A patient with capacity can also consciously choose to refuse food and fluids. The decision to stop eating and drinking is legally and ethically indistinguishable from the informed choice to refuse any other forms of life-sustaining treatment. VSED is an informed choice for a patient with a prognosis of weeks or months, rather than imminently dying, as is generally required for palliative sedation.[15]

VSED is a patient's informed choice. It has the advantage of not requiring a physician's order. Quill and Byock suggest that: "In practice, honoring the decision requires the support of the family, physician, and health care team, who must provide appropriate palliative care as the dying process unfolds."[16] A patient choosing VSED will not normally complain of hunger or thirst but may experience symptoms such as agitation or delirium as the dying process unfolds. Under these conditions, palliative sedation may be required.

Patients who choose VSED die of dehydration, generally, not starvation. Terminal dehydration is considered one of the best ways to die and most hospice caregivers rate it as a very comfortable death. Dehydration has an analgesic effect and leads to a decrease in sensation and awareness. Thirst, pain, and nausea are actually rare symptoms in death by dehydration. A dry mouth is a common symptom but can be alleviated with mouth swabs.

In Oregon, where physician-assisted suicide has been legal for decades, the rate of death by choosing VSED is, among hospice patients, quite high. Most of the choices for VSED were not made because the patient was experiencing intolerable physical symptoms; according to the hospice nurses who accompanied the VSED patients on their path: "[Patients] chose to stop eating and drinking for reasons that included being ready to die, believing that continuing to live was pointless, and a sense of poor quality of life, as well as wanting to control the manner of death. Unbearable physical suffering did not appear to be an important reason for this choice."[17]

Because VSED is a patient's informed choice, trying to force food, fluid or providing artificial nutrition and hydration necessarily violates the patient's informed choice. Such actions would be a battery under common law and could well be prosecutable. Dying under VSED can take days or several weeks depending on the patient's symptom-burden and medical condition at the outset.[18]

If a patient who chooses VSED loses capacity and experiences hallucinations or delirium during the dying process, she may request food or fluids. Typically, the patient requests a specific food or fluid. It is Quill's and Byock's recommendation to offer the requested food or fluid. They also recommend that, if the request persists, the VSED plan should be reevaluated.[19] However, if the plan is reevaluated due to the patient's delirium, it may be that we have violated the patient's informed choice for VSED when he had proper capacity. If the patient experiences delirium during the dying process, he has by definition lost decision-making capacity. It becomes unclear which request we should honor. Moreover, if the patient's delirium persists, then terminal sedation may be appropriate.[20] In Oregon, 12.5 percent of patients who chose VSED resumed eating and drinking "most often because of thirst or pressure from family members."[21]

If the patient is living with a quality of life that is unacceptable to him or her due to existential suffering, the choice for VSED should be explored more closely. It may be that VSED is wholly inappropriate for patients living with fear, guilt or shame. Sometimes fear and guilt, if not shame, are appropriate and cannot be relieved by the interdisciplinary team, including the medical social worker or the chaplain. In that case, VSED may become appropriate once all other interventions have been tried and failed. VSED may also be appropriate for an elderly patient with chronic illness who is just "tired of life."

The choice for VSED needs to be both informed and free. The patient's mental and emotional health should always be assessed to make certain that the choice for VSED is not due to unrecognized and treatable depression or anxiety. Contrast the cases of patients suffering from anorexia nervosa or clinical depression—in these cases the refusal of food and fluids is a symptom and not a free choice.

An exceptionally important distinction to understand is that when the choice for VSED is free and informed, that choice is *not suicide*. It is ethically and legally equivalent to refusing life-sustaining treatment. "In contrast, for a patient with severe, unrelieved suffering and advanced, incurable illness, cessation of eating and drinking might be considered part of the right to refuse treatment."[22]

Rather than supporting a patient who chooses VSED, physicians and nurses are of course free to refuse for reasons of conscience. In that event, the objecting physician or nurse is obligated to find healthcare professionals who will support the patient during the dying process. Otherwise:

> An absolute stance (refusal) of this nature creates a double bind for patients who are ready for death and desire the continued help of their physician. If such patients are honest about their intention, their request for physician support cannot be granted. To maintain a therapeutic relationship and be guaranteed continued symptom management, they and their families may have to collude in a deception and conceal their decision to stop eating and drinking.[23]

Case 13-2. Going Backward.

Kitty Lennon is a thirty-four-year-old patient with metastatic lung cancer. She is on home hospice but she feels that she is just dying too slowly. Kitty states she wants to get her dying process "over with".

Kitty has decision-making capacity and makes an informed choice for VSED. Five days later she has become confused and now lacks decision-making capacity. She calls out for water which is given to her with sips off a spoon. As the days go on and her dying process continues, Kitty experiences delirium and agitation. She is given morphine and Ativan. She dies a week later.

Discussion Questions

- Kitty clearly asked for water. Did Kitty have the capacity to make a decision to stop VSED? Or should we not give her the water, as she made a conscious choice to start VSED?

- As Kitty dies, experiencing delirium and agitation, should we medicate her, or give her intravenous hydration?

Case 13-3. A Choice.

Georgia Ellison is an eighty-three-year-old patient with uterine cancer that has metastasized throughout her pelvic area. Her physician informs Georgia that there is no effective treatment and he recommends hospice. Georgia states: "I'm not ready for that yet." Georgia lives at an assisted living retirement home with her husband of sixty years, Fred. Georgia is living with a quality of life that is satisfying to her.

When Fred dies, Georgia's medical condition and her quality of life decline rapidly and she opts for hospice. She remains in her retirement home. Georgia's pain is well managed, but she begins to have diarrhea and humiliating "accidents." As a result, Georgia stays in her room, refusing to go downstairs to the main dining room where she used to socialize with friends and the other residents. Georgia's meals are brought to her room, but she eats very little and loses thirty pounds. Her friends in the retirement home are worried about her and frequently stop by Georgia's room to check up on her. Georgia turns them away every time and they soon learn to leave her alone.

Georgia is not dying as quickly as she would like. Her eyesight is compromised, and she can no longer read, her favorite activity. Georgia's quality of life is rapidly becoming intolerable to her although her pain is well managed. Georgia feels that her dying process is being prolonged and she wants to hasten her death.

Georgia asks the hospice nurse and the chaplain about assisted suicide but they tell her that assisted suicide is illegal in her state of residence. They offer palliative sedation when her death is imminent, but they refuse to give her extra medication that will hasten her death. Georgia then begins to hoard pills, taking less medication than prescribed and suffering moderate pain as a result.

Georgia's prognosis is measured in months, not weeks. The hospice team believes that giving Georgia palliative sedation when she is not imminently dying is unethical. They also have concerns that Georgia's suffering is more existential than physical. However, Georgia simply does not want to wait. Her existential, emotional, and spiritual suffering (and her fear of physical suffering) have become intolerable to her.

Georgia contemplates refusing food and fluids in order to hasten her death. She explores this idea with her hospice nurse and the hospice chaplain. They explain to her that voluntarily stopping eating and drinking (VSED) is an ethical and legal option for her and that the hospice team will support her if she makes this choice. Georgia agrees to be evaluated for an affective disorder, including clinical depression and suicidal ideation, prior to beginning her fast. She passes the assessment and is determined to have a high level of decision-making capacity.

Georgia remains awake, alert, and symptom-free for the first four days of her fast. Then she slips into a coma. She dies ten days after beginning VSED.

Discussion Questions

- Are the hospice nurse and chaplain wrong to support Georgia's choice as she still has such a long time to live? If not, what support should they give?

- Is Georgia's life intolerable to her or is she being impatient?

- Should we be surprised if Georgia takes her hoarded pills? What if she becomes comatose but does not die?

Chapter 14. The Principle of Double Effect

Case 14-1. A Dying Cancer Patient with Pain.

Katy Lamb is a thirty-year-old patient dying from uterine cancer with metastasis to the bone, liver, and brain. She is suffering from intolerable and intractable pain. She has the capacity to make an informed choice to receive comfort medications only and her loved ones agree. She wants to remain as aware as possible so that she can enjoy visits from her family. Therefore, palliative sedation is not an option. Katy chooses to be admitted to hospice so that her symptoms can be managed and her quality of life can be maintained until her death.

Then Katy's pain becomes intolerable. She tells her hospice nurse that her pain "is a fifteen out of ten." Soon, she enters the active dying phase of her disease and becomes minimally responsive, responding only with signs of pain when she is repositioned. Her loved ones gather around her and pour out tearful expressions of love and gratitude for what she means to them.

The increasing doses of opioids required to alleviate Katy's pain run the risk of depressing her respiratory drive and hastening her death. Her family knows this. They collectively decide that Katy should be made comfortable and her dying process should not be prolonged.

Discussion Questions

- Is it right to give so much medication that we eliminate Katy's pain and hasten her death?

- If we eliminate Katy's pain and thereby hasten her death, are we killing her? Or are we letting her die?

- **What are the alternatives to aggressive management of Katy's pain?**

A dying patient has a *right* to be free from physical suffering. Intolerable pain, anxiety, dyspnea, seizures, and other physical suffering must be eliminated whenever possible. Where palliative sedation is not an option, then high dosages of opioids, benzodiazepines, or other medications may be necessary. Very high doses of opioids in a patient with opioid tolerance are generally non-controversial. However, sometimes the level of medication necessary to reduce suffering to tolerable levels may depress respiratory drive. Medications can usually be increased to tolerable levels without the risk of hastening death. However, there are some cases where physical suffering is intolerable with the usual levels of medication. In these cases, the level of medication must be increased to a level that risks depressing respiratory drive and hastening death. "Physicians have an obligation to relieve pain and suffering and to promote the dignity and autonomy of dying patients in their care. This includes providing effective palliative treatment even though it may foreseeably hasten death."[1]

When a patient, his surrogate decision-maker, or his family has made an informed choice for palliative treatment the physician, save for reasons of conscience, *must honor* that choice. Part of honoring that informed choice is accepting the risk of hastened death as part of the promise to relieve suffering. Ethics and the law both honor this commitment. A physician is justified when she orders a level of medication that hastens death. If the patient's suffering is intolerable and intractable at lower levels, higher doses of medication are ethically necessary. The physician is justified in giving the necessary medication by the principle of double effect.

The *principle of double effect,* first developed by Thomas Aquinas, is applied to conflict situations. In a conflict situation, any action will result in numerous effects, both good and bad. In its traditional form, the principle of double effect has four conditions:

- The act must not be evil; it must be good in and of itself or, at the very least, indifferent.

- The intended good effect must not be the result of the bad effect.

- The bad effect must not be intended in itself, only permitted or foreseen.

- There must be proportionately grave reason for permitting the bad effect.

In a more modern definition, the principle of double effect will justify an action with multiple effects if:

- The actor does not intend the bad effect, either as end or means.

- There is proportionate reason for allowing the bad effect.[2]

The test case for the principle of double effect is a dying patient who requires heavy doses of opioids to relieve intolerable suffering and terminal sedation is not available:

- The "camera picture" of the act of giving the medication is a good act, or at least indifferent.

- The good of alleviating suffering is not the result of hastening death. We are not alleviating the patient's death by relieving them of his or her life, as we would in euthanasia.

- We do not intend to hasten death. We intend to alleviate intolerable and intractable suffering. The hastening of death is a foreseeable consequence but is not intended.

- A grave reason for hastening the patient's death is the patient's intolerable suffering. A physician is justified to order high levels of medication if necessary, to bring the patient's suffering to a tolerable level. The use of medication is a proportionate reason for permitting the hastening of the patient's death.

In short, without the justification of the principle of double effect, many dying patients would suffer needlessly.

Case 14-2. Hastening Death by Removing a Ventilator.

Jim Joyce, a sixty-one-year-old man, is dying from multi-system organ failure and is dependent upon a ventilator. He has the capacity to request comfort measures only and that the ventilator be withdrawn. However, as the ventilator is withdrawn, he is frightened that he will experience suffocation.

Once the ventilator is withdrawn, Jim does in fact require increasing amounts of sedatives to avoid the subjective experience of suffocation. His physician sees a blurred line between the respiratory distress due to the ventilator being withdrawn, allowing the patient to die, and the high levels of medication necessary to relieve Jim's feeling of suffocation. Jim's physician understands that she may order medication that will hasten Jim's death as they further depress his respiratory drive.

Discussion Questions

- **Are we killing Jim by eliminating his feelings of suffocation?**
- **Is there an alternative?**

Chapter 15. Physician-Assisted Suicide

Case 15-1. The Case of Kenneth Bergstedt.

Kenneth was a thirty-year-old Nevada man with quadriplegia. He wanted to be allowed to die because his father, who cared for him, was himself dying of cancer. Kenneth, though not in physical pain, feared he would be institutionalized without his father's support. A psychiatric evaluation submitted to the trial court found that Kenneth was depressed but that this was irrelevant because "the quality of life for this man is forever profaned by a future which offers no relief and only the possibility of worsening."

Based on his poor quality of life the Nevada Supreme Court upheld Kenneth's decision to die. No consideration was given to promoting Kenneth's quality of life and human dignity—such as a non-institutional, in-home health care option. A dissenting Nevada Supreme Court Justice observed that: "[w]ith this kind of support it is no wonder that he decided to do himself in."[1]

The terminology must be crystal clear in any discussion about physician-assisted suicide.

Euthanasia is the act of a physician killing a patient who is suffering intolerable and intractable symptoms for reasons of mercy and compassion—a mercy killing. Generally, the patent dies after being injected with opioids or potassium chloride. The physician ends the patient's suffering by ending the patient's life.

In *physician-assisted suicide*, the physician writes a prescription, generally for barbiturates. The patient, not the physician, will administer the lethal dose of the medication. Physician-assisted suicide is, of course, a last-resort option. It is ethical only if all other reasonable means of eliminating the patient's suffering have been tried and failed. In physician-assisted suicide, the physician intends the death of the patient, also for reasons of mercy and compassion. However, in physician-assisted suicide, *the patient is the agent.* The physician signs a prescription, a slip of paper, and hands it to the patient. The patient's will and intention alone commit him to swallowing the pills.

The intentions are different in withholding and withdrawing life-sustaining treatment, palliative sedation, the principle of double effect, and physician-assisted suicide. In all four, we intend to relieve the patient's intolerable and intractable suffering.

- In withdrawing and withholding life-sustaining treatment, we foresee and allow, but do not intend, the death of the patient.

- In palliative sedation, we use medications to end the patient's suffering.

- When medications are prescribed to alleviate intolerable and intractable suffering, the principle of double effect safeguards is that we foresee and allow, but do not intend, the death of the patient.

In all four, the patient's underlying fatal pathology is the legal and ethical cause of death. Physician-assisted suicide is different. We intend the death of the patient.

Physician-assisted suicide is simple for the physician who evaluates the patient and the level of suffering and writes a prescription. The act of withdrawing a ventilator, for example, requires much more of the physician.

Like voluntarily stopping eating and drinking, the patient choosing physician-assisted suicide requires a high level of decision-making capacity. It is, after all, a decision for death. The decision must be made by the patient himself. A patient's surrogate may decide to withhold or withdraw life-sustaining treatment, consent to palliative sedation, or administer medications according to the principle of double effect, but she cannot choose physician-assisted suicide.

In physician-assisted suicide, the patient generally dies before death is naturally imminent—*imminence of death* is generally defined as fourteen days without extraordinary measures. Palliative sedation is far less controversial a subject when death is already imminent. In physician-assisted suicide, the patient may take the fatal medication at any point during his terminal illness, defined as a prognosis of six months or less.

In physician-assisted suicide, the physician's intention is the death of the patient by prescribing drugs, though the medication will be taken and swallowed by the patient without the participation of anyone else. The patient's cause of death is *external* to the patient. The motive is the same in all five practices—compassion—but the *intentions* are different. It may be that the patient requests physician-assisted suicide because of intolerable suffering from the underlying fatal pathology. However, the chain of causation between the fatal pathology and the patient's death is attenuated.

Arguments Supporting Physician-Assisted Suicide.

The duty to respect individual autonomy is the major argument for physician-assisted suicide. Proponents argue that there is a duty to respect patient self-determination absolutely. A patient's decision to hasten his death, in order to protect his personal values, is a deeply personal exercise of self-determination. It does not impair the rights of anyone else or incur any other social cost—in fact, quite the opposite.

Proponents argue that the patient's request for lethal medication may be the only way of maintaining a measure of control over our personal death in the modern world. Society must allow a terminally ill and suffering patient to end her life with dignity—on her own terms. We cannot withhold the only option that this patient has to escape his suffering without interference by others. Peter Singer stated that making people die the way that we want them to die is the most "odious form of tyranny."[2] To force a person to endure the unendurable is the mark of torture, not medicine.

The *Philosophers' Brief* (the amicus brief filed by five bioethicist professors in *Washington v Glucksberg* and *Vacco v Quill*) states:

> The humaneness of a death is not only a matter of avoiding pain and physical suffering; it is also a matter of consonance with a patient's most basic values. For some patients, a death softened by the heavy use of painkillers or hastened by withholding or withdrawing life-sustaining treatment will be tolerable; for others such prospects are profoundly repugnant: these patients fear and resent a death preceded by a period of obtundation, or in which their bodies slowly deteriorate from the ravages of a lethal disease. Not all patients will choose to die in the same way, even when death is imminent: some will prefer continued aggressive treatment, in the hope that they can beat the odds; some will prefer withdrawing or withholding specific forms of treatment; others will accept death as a consequence of escalating doses of morphine; still others will choose to forego nutrition and hydration; some will tolerate terminal sedation; but some strongly prefer a peaceful and humane death directly initiated

while conscious and alert, facilitated by the assistance of a physician.[3]

Quill and Byock argue that requests for physician-assisted suicide are infrequently triggered by unrelieved pain alone. The requests generally result from "a combination of physical symptoms and debility, weakness, lack of meaning, and weariness of dying."[4] Usually, the suffering of a patient requesting lethal medication is "a complex amalgam of pain; physical symptoms; and psychosocial, existential, and spiritual issues, which are balanced by hope, love, connection, and meaning." Suffering can also arise from the threat of the disintegration of the patient, as he knows himself, or a loss of meaning in life. Quill and Byock argue that good palliative medicine requires understanding and responding to each patient's unique suffering.[5] The loss of autonomy, the fear of losing autonomy, and perceived feelings of being a burden, are cited as the principal reasons that patients want to hasten their deaths.[6]

In Oregon, where physician-assisted suicide has been legal since 1997, the three most frequently mentioned end-of-life concerns expressed by patients who choose physician-assisted suicide are: a loss of autonomy, a decreasing ability to participate in activities that make life enjoyable, and the loss of their personal dignity. Burden on family, friends and caregivers is cited by almost half of patients. Fear of pain and financial implications of treatment together were cited in only about 30 percent of the cases.[7]

Carl Wellman wrote:

> Why does it matter whether or not one dies with dignity? It is important to the patient because when and how one dies profoundly affects the meaning of one's death and, thus, the shape and significance of one's life. One's life is a

biography experienced as a drama with a beginning, a middle, and an end such that the intrinsic value of each part is determined much more by one's awareness of its significance for the whole than by its felt pleasantness or painfulness. The awareness that one will die without dignity can undermine one's self-respect and cause one to devalue one's life. The loss of a patient's dignity also affects how others remember her and reduces, at least to some degree, their respect for her. This is an injury to the patient, who must now expect to be remembered less fondly and with less respect than she would wish, and a misfortune to friends and family members, who are condemned to live on with distressful memories of the death of their loved one.[8]

Anecdotal evidence shows that the grief of a family whose loved one "died with dignity" is less painful, less traumatic, and more coherent.

Most terminally ill patients are reassured that they can end their lives if their suffering becomes intractable and intolerable, but the vast majority will never need to hasten their deaths. Where physician-assisted suicide is not legal, patients—even families—may hoard pills in case of unrelieved suffering. Patients may commit suicide without medical help, or loved ones and physicians may wish to "put the patient out of their suffering."

Quill has stated:

> I have, under duress, used terminal sedation and withdrawal of foods and fluids for the hastening of death to relieve terminal suffering when these were the only available options. I have also assisted suicide by lethal oral barbiturates and can categorically say that there is no

comparison in the quality and dignity of death as far as the patient and her family are concerned. The former methods may preserve the "moral" and legal integrity of the physician, but they do not serve the best interests of the patient and her family.[9]

A lethal dose of barbiturates allows the patient to die with dignity and is "without futility or hypocrisy."[10]

Proponents of physician-assisted suicide also argue that, outside the states where physician-assisted suicide is legal, there is a secret practice of physician-assisted death (and euthanasia). Patients, loved ones, and physicians will all wish to hasten death in order to respect a patient's wish to die or because of observable, unrelenting symptoms. However, where there is secrecy there are no safeguards.

The secret practice of hastened death is, of course, extremely difficult to study. A physician admitting participation—or even knowledge—is admitting to a crime, and along with any family present, runs the risk of prosecution. On the other hand, it appears that district attorneys have little interest in prosecuting such cases providing they are not blatant. This leads to a "don't ask, don't tell" situation and as we have seen, such situations are highly subject to abuse. If the practice of physician-assisted suicide is secret, then there is no documentation to be reviewed and there are no consultations required from physicians experienced in hospice and palliative care. In essence, we lose all potential scientific knowledge—and commensurate benefit to patients—by preferring to keep our institutional head in the sand.

Before physician-assisted suicide was legal in any state, Timothy Quill admitted in the New England Journal of Medicine that he assisted a middle-aged woman diagnosed with acute myelogenous leukemia to commit suicide. He used the pseudonym Diane. Diane refused chemotherapy for her condition. Quill stated that Diane was well aware that she would certainly die without treatment. She was upset by her diagnosis but was not terribly depressed. Diane well understood that her death would likely be painful and prolonged; she requested a supply of barbiturates, ostensibly as sleeping pills. Quill made certain that Diane knew how many barbiturates she needed to sleep and how many barbiturates she needed to die. Quill provided the prescription as well as directions for its use. Diane took her life.[11] Quill was never prosecuted. Other physicians were doing the same thing at the time. For example, in 1995 in the State of Washington, twelve percent of physicians polled reported that they had been asked by their terminally ill patients for prescriptions to hasten death, and of these, twenty-four percent had complied with the request.[12]

In 2016, California adopted the End of Life Option Act (commonly known as the "EOLOA") which contains many of the safeguards instituted by the older Oregon Death with Dignity Act, enacted in 1997; however, the EOLOA is much more comprehensive. Until the EOLOA, the Oregon Act was the model for other states where physician-assisted suicide is legal.

Under the EOLOA, *informed decision* means a decision by a patient with a terminal diagnosis who has the following information:

- The patient's diagnosis and prognosis, as confirmed by a second physician.

- The potential risks associated with taking the "aid-in-dying" drug to be prescribed.

- The probable result of taking the drug to be prescribed.

- The possibility that the individual may choose not to obtain the drug or may obtain the drug but may decide not to ingest it.

- The feasible alternatives or additional treatment opportunities, including, but not limited to, comfort care and pain management, palliative care, and hospice care.

The prescribing physician must confirm that the patient's decision is not coerced or influenced by having a private conversation with the patient alone. The physician must also inform the patient that he may withdraw or rescind the request for an aid-in-dying drug at any time and in any manner. The physician must allow the patient every opportunity to change his mind before prescribing the aid-in-dying drug. Finally, depression not affecting decision-making capacity is not a bar to receiving the prescription for the aid-in-dying drug. By law, assisted death is not indicated as suicide on the patient's death certificate.

The purpose of the EOLOA , and similar acts in other states, is to offer the dying patient "a humane and dignified" death. To this end, the first form that the patient must fill out is titled: REQUEST FOR AN AID-IN-DYING DRUG TO END MY LIFE IN A HUMANE AND DIGNIFIED MANNER. The second form, to be filled out within forty-eight hours of the physician writing the prescription is titled: FINAL ATTESTATION FOR AN AID-IN-DYING DRUG TO END MY LIFE IN A HUMANE AND DIGNIFIED MANNER. The attending and consulting physicians must also fill out forms.

In the states that have legalized physician-assisted suicide, reasons cited for requesting the lethal medication include:

- The decreasing ability to participate in activities that made life enjoyable

- The loss of control of bodily functions

- Persistent and uncontrollable pain and suffering
- A loss of dignity

Yet, any or all of these types of suffering are reasonable responses to a terminal illness and to the harms associated with the treatments for a terminal illness.

If a patient selects physician-assisted suicide because of the fear of "persistent and uncontrollable pain and suffering" we must wonder if some terminally ill patients do not trust their physicians to relieve their symptoms. Despite efforts at education, some physicians still undertreat pain because of the fear that a terminally ill patient will become addicted. Perhaps we need to recall our foremost promise to the patient that we will treat relentless pain and suffering.

The American public largely supports physician-assisted suicide and euthanasia.[13] Americans generally favor allowing doctors to assist terminally ill patients in ending their lives but the degree of support ranges from 51 percent to 70 percent, depending on how the process is described. A 2013 Gallup Poll showed that 70 percent of Americans are in favor of euthanasia in limited circumstances, when physicians hasten a terminally ill patient's death and the action is described as allowing doctors to "end the patient's life by some painless means." However, only 51 percent support physician-assisted suicide when the process is described as doctors helping a patient to "commit suicide" - a variance which is probably due to the societal stigma associated with suicide. A wording that refers to the patient's intention to end his life as "suicide" connotes that the patient is alone and others are not involved in the decision, nor does it specify that the procedure will involve painless and compassionate means. This use of phrasing, and the traditional discomfort with suicide, appears to account for the lower approval rate.

For many proponents, however, the argument goes further. Presently, physician-assisted suicide requires that the patient be physically capable of self-administering and swallowing the lethal amount of medication. Proponents of extending the right insist that we should provide euthanasia for patients who cannot self-administer drugs, thereby allowing patients to enjoy lives with reasonable quality of life as long as is possible. When a patient asks to die, the euthanasia is "voluntary."

However, some patients do not possess the capacity to ask for voluntary euthanasia. Proponents state that we might use substituted judgment or best-interests arguments to euthanize patients who lack decision-making capacity. This is called *nonvoluntary euthanasia*. Persistent vegetative state and end-stage dementia patients would be candidates for nonvoluntary euthanasia as many people, including their decision-makers, may view either condition as "a fate worse than death." In coming years, it might even be possible to request euthanasia in advance in a detailed advance directive.

However, we do not *need* to euthanize persistent vegetative state and end-stage dementia patients. We can allow them to die comfortably by withdrawing or withholding artificial nutrition and hydration.

Proponents of physician-assisted suicide also argue that the right should be possessed by all patients who are enduring intolerable, unrelievable suffering of any kind. We should not limit physician-assisted suicide to patients who are terminally ill from a physiological illness—this is, frankly, *cruel*. We should extend physician-assisted suicide to patients enduring intolerable and unrelievable suffering resulting from chronic and psychiatric diseases. The rationale here is that we cannot deny the *right to die* to chronically ill patients who will suffer longer than terminally ill patients will, nor can we deny the right to die comfortably and effectively with physician assistance to patients suffering with mental disorders where psychotropic medication does not work.

Proponents of the right to physician-assisted suicide also argue from the *principle of equal protection*. This states that Justice requires that we treat like cases alike; we must provide the same rights to similarly situated patients. Terminally ill patients with capacity are allowed to hasten death by refusing life-sustaining treatment. However, for some patients with capacity who are not dependent on life-sustaining technologies, refusal of treatment will not hasten death. The only option for these patients is physician-assisted suicide. The mandate of Justice then requires that we should allow it for them. This argument was made before the United States Supreme Court in *Vacco v. Quill*. It failed.

It may be that a patient who fears the decline of his quality of life may take the lethal medication *before* his quality of life becomes unacceptable and he can no longer swallow. The fear of losing the ability to swallow may force a patient to take the pills while he still can. A patient who may have a quality of life that is otherwise acceptable to him might wish to make certain to die before his quality of life declines. This patient may die earlier than he may wish because–according to the standing law–he must be able to swallow the pills.

Another strong proponent position is that the physician has the *duty* to relieve the patient's suffering. *Physician-assisted suicide is an act of mercy and compassion*. If a patient asks for a promise from the physician to assist in his death when his suffering becomes intolerable, then trust is fundamentally eroded when physician-assisted suicide is not even an option. A patient may mistrust that the physician will treat extreme suffering at the end of life. When physician-assisted suicide is not legal, the physician is essentially abandoning the patient.

At the time that the Supreme Court was considering two physician-assisted suicide cases, Quill stated that, although not all terminally ill patients want physician-assisted suicide, most want it as a backup plan should suffering become intolerable. "Those patients who do not choose to exercise their right to physician-assisted suicide may gain comfort in the knowledge that the option exists if their suffering becomes intolerable. For many, this will make it possible to live fuller, more complete lives during the process of dying, since they need not fear a bad death."[14] "I think a considerable number of people . . . would seek some reassurance from their doctor that, `Gee, if things get really horrible, will you be there for me.' That's the fundamental commitment that I believe we should be making."[15]

Arguments against Legalization of Physician-Assisted Suicide

Opponents of the right to physician-assisted suicide most often argue from a religious or secular humanist view of the value of human life. It is of course true that there are strong religious and secular humanist traditions against taking human life—rightly so. Opponents of physician-assisted suicide argue that physician-assisted suicide is morally wrong because it contradicts these beliefs and endangers the value that our society places on life.

Opponents to the right of physician-assisted suicide also argue that there is no duty to respect autonomy absolutely. If a patient does not get everything he wants with regard to futile treatment, then nor should a patient get everything he wants with regard to hastening death. The core argument here is that autonomy is not self-justifying. They hold that the right to have help in killing oneself or the right to be killed is not a basic human need and therefore we do not need to provide it.

The historical and ethical traditions of medicine are generally opposed to ending a patient's life. There are, however, many versions of the Hippocratic Oath. One states: "I will not administer poison to anyone where asked." The American Medical Association and other professional groups officially oppose physician-assisted suicide.[16] However, as the California End of Life Option Act was being discussed in the state legislature, the California Medical Association withdrew its historical objections and took a neutral stance—a truly demonstrative step.[17]

The American Medical Association's primary opposition to physician-assisted suicide is based on a concern that linking physician-assisted suicide to the practice of medicine will harm the public's image of the profession. Physician-assisted suicide is: "fundamentally incompatible with the physician's role as healer, would be difficult or impossible to control, and would pose serious societal risks."[18] "Physicians must not perform euthanasia or participate in assisted suicide . . . In certain carefully defined circumstances, it would be humane to recognize that death is certain and suffering is great. However, the societal risks of involving physicians in medical interventions to cause patients' deaths is too great to condone euthanasia or physician-assisted suicide at this time."[19] The American Medical Association instead encourages respect, communication, and adequate pain management.

The National Hospice and Palliative Care Organization (NHPCO) does not support the legalization of physician-assisted suicide— however, the lay of the land is evolving and they recognize this fact. The NHPCO states in its resolution on physician-assisted suicide that it is committed to the value of life: "Our society's ability to meet the comprehensive needs of patients with life-limiting illnesses and their family members (from day-to-day caregiving through bereavement) are severely deficient. The work that must be done in the areas of professional education, public awareness, healthcare systems development, alignment of financial driving forces, public policy revision to eliminate barriers and promote best practices, and research to increase the fund of knowledge needed to improve care, is monumental."[20]

Relentless pain is generally not the reason why patients request physician-assisted suicide and other means of hastening death. Generally, a dying person requests hastened death due to a wide range of suffering, such as:

- Physical symptoms other than pain such as weakness and frailty
- Inability to concentrate
- No enjoyment in formerly enjoyable activities
- A perceived feeling of being burdensome to and dependent on others
- Depression and/or anxiety
- Senses of helplessness and/or hopelessness
- Loss of meaning in life

In order to decrease the number of requests for physician-assisted suicide, we need to address not only the terminally ill patient's physical symptoms but the emotional, spiritual, and relational situation. Adrienne Asch writes:

> When these data reveal that fear of burdening others is of much greater concern to patients who seek suicide than concerns about finances or physical pain, then how can professionals and families know that the supposedly autonomous wish to end life is not a response to a patient's deep fear that she has become disliked, distasteful to, and resented by the very people from whom

she seeks expertise, physical help, and emotional
support?[21]

Opponents of physician-assisted suicide argue that if physician-assisted suicide were legalized for patients other than the terminally ill, the most vulnerable members of society would be affected. Physician-assisted suicide for the disabled, for example, would result in further prejudice against persons who are already discounted by society. It is important to remember that the Nazis began the holocaust by systematically killing Germans with disabilities.

A valid oppositional concern here is that mainstream society *already* stereotypes its most vulnerable members. The demented and mentally ill, the elderly, and the disabled are believed by some to be "unproductive" to society at large. The poor (and ethnic and racial minorities) already face discrimination in the availability of medical services. Some might believe themselves to be "humane" when they eliminate people who are not "whole" or "not there"—they are not.

Disabled persons in particular face internalized stigma, social oppression, and a disgraceful paucity of the social services required for them to live full and rewarding lives. All too often, those who are "not us" are not those who live worthwhile lives–as "we" do. Disability rights activists point out that many newly disabled persons are incorrectly believed to be terminally ill–also pointing out that the terminally ill are disabled.

Disability rights activists fear that a public policy of physician-assisted suicide will threaten the lives of disabled persons who are not terminally ill. The fact is, many disabled people have internalized negative social stigmas and view themselves as burdensome. Vulnerable people, the argument goes, may be pushed into physician-assisted suicide because they may lack access to social services and the things that make life worth living. Burdened family members and healthcare providers may encourage physician-assisted suicide for the disabled. Alternatively, some suggest it might be even more compassionate to inform a disabled person of the right to physician-assisted suicide. Once again, one area that none of us, from the greatest institutions to the single medical practitioner, can think to supplant is the singular right of self-determination—regardless of the complexity of the surrounding arguments.

For these reasons, most disability rights activists are concerned with life-ending decisions for vulnerable persons. Again, Adrienne Asch writes:

> Once the severely disabled, ill, or dying person is seen as "other"—as different, not quite in the human and moral community, even past friendship and familial bonds— social bonds can diminish. To anyone with the capacity to perceive the difference between warmth, toleration, and coldness in how he is treated by others, the thought of days, months, or years of life subject to resentful, duty-filled physical ministrations may be a fate worse than death, akin to imprisonment and solitary confinement.[22]

Diane Coleman, the former president of Not Dead Yet, a disability rights advocacy organization, stated in a Congressional hearing: "Here's how I'm beginning to look at things. The far right wants to kill us slowly and painfully by cutting the things we need to live, health care, public housing and transportation, etc. The far left wants to kill us quickly and call it compassion, while also saving money for others perhaps deemed more worthy."[23] Diane Coleman said that the prejudice with which the able-bodied community believed that Terri Schiavo's life was "worse than death"–thus supporting the withdrawal of her artificial nutrition and hydration—was the "tip of a very large and almost fully submerged iceberg."[24]

Disability rights activists also argue, however, that the most severe disability does not diminish the experiential worth of a life. Although it is difficult to suggest that physical misery, social barriers, and lifelong prejudices don't diminish the experience of life, the real core of the problem *here* is prejudice, negative and inaccurate stereotypes, and most of all—societal indifference.[25]

Not Dead Yet, writing in opposition to the California End of Life Option Act, states:

> The bill specifically provides that depression is not a barrier to getting a lethal prescription. All that is required is that the depression is viewed as not impairing the person's judgment, a subjective and speculative assessment at best. Psychiatrists and psychologists are not immune from prevailing social biases against people whose illnesses make them dependent on others for basic physical care. In some cases, they are just as likely as anyone to say, "If I were in your shoes, I might want to die," and render an opinion that treatment for depression is not necessary, paving the way for a lethal solution.[26]

We can clearly see that opponents of physician-assisted suicide primarily fear that the terminally ill and the disabled will eventually feel that they have a *duty* to die. In general, we believe that there is a higher duty to live than to die but that intuition may become inverted for the vulnerable. Debilitated patients already *carry* the burden of *being* a burden, long before an "inversion of values." Taken in a different light, the duty to compassionately end life might seem the only course of action compatible with human dignity and human worth.

If a state overtly excluded people with "terminal" disabilities from suicide prevention laws and programs, it would undoubtedly violate federal civil rights laws . . . Yet that is precisely the design and effect of the Oregon assisted-suicide law. A more devastating form of discrimination would be difficult to imagine. By assuming that it is irrational for a non-disabled person to end his life, but rational for a disabled person to do so, the law assumes that the non-disabled person's life is intrinsically more valuable and worthwhile than that of a disabled person. . . Central to this movement is the idea that a disabling condition does not inherently diminish one's life; rather, surrounding barriers and prejudices do so. Assisted suicide takes the opposite approach—it gives official sanction to the idea that life with a disabling condition is not worth living.[27]

It is completely natural for a patient with a protracted illness to fear being a burden on family caregivers. Family caregivers frequently must quit work, expend all their savings and subsequently suffer financial hardship—as just one example. Many become physically and emotionally exhausted. There may be family tension and latent guilt about placing the patient in a skilled nursing facility. Family caregivers are frequently demoralized and depressed. The feeling of being a burden, and the wish to spare her family, is not an undue influence on an *informed choice* for physician-assisted suicide. A patient might reasonably find that a "good death" is preferable to burdening her caregivers.

We have to understand that some members of vulnerable populations already mistrust the medical establishment. "The lived experience of the poor and marginalized may ground a more general distrust of the medical profession and of the value that society attaches to their lives."[28] It is well known that patients from vulnerable groups, age, race, ethnicity, and gender are less likely to be assessed for pain and when assessed are less likely to receive pain medication.[29] The infamous Tuskegee syphilis study is not far from the minds of some African American patients and their families. Wealthy people fear overtreatment. Vulnerable people receive undertreatment.

Physician-assisted suicide may become a cost-containment strategy because it is cheaper than providing medical or social services. Anecdotal evidence shows that health insurers in Oregon have been known to send letters to terminally ill patients advising them of their "right" to physician-assisted suicide. The insurers may or may not cover the cost of the lethal medication. Barbiturates are cheap. The cost of a lethal dose of Seconal is less than $200 online. Because of the conflict of interest, the California law prevents insurers from informing their insureds about the option of physician-assisted suicide.

Disability rights advocates state that they are denied approval for basic medical services because the treatments will not "cure" the disabled patient. The costs are too high to provide treatment and social services to people who have been cast aside.

> The idea of mixing a cost-cutting "treatment" such as assisted suicide into a cost-conscious health care system that's poorly designed to meet a seriously ill patient's needs is dangerous to the thousands of people whose health care costs the most—mainly people living with a disability, the elderly and chronically ill.[30]

Opponents of the right to physician-assisted suicide, like the American Medical Association, argue that extending the legal right to physician-assisted suicide will destroy public trust in the medical profession. The fear is that the power imbalance between physician and patient will cause a patient to choose physician-assisted suicide in order to please the physician. There will be no hope of *informed choice* because of the patient's compulsion to consent to the physician's perceived demands or the fear that the physician will abandon him or her. A patient may fear a physician who holds the power of death in her hands. A patient may fear that his over-worked physician regards him or her as a burden; a patient may feel that the physician wants him to die and get it over with. Even if the physician is careful not to *recommend* physician-assisted suicide, her patient may not hear that there is a choice. The legalization of physician-assisted suicide will further imbalance the power between physician and patient. Physicians are highly educated, tend to be wealthier, and upper class; patients frequently are not. The power differential may impair a patient's ability to choose freely between physician-assisted suicide and living out his illness to natural death.

Further, because of the difference in power, the physician's presentation of the option for assisted suicide may be heard as a recommendation. A patient may "go along" with what he perceives as the physician's recommendation, rather than choose from a genuine desire of his own. The theoretical danger here is that any discussion in which the physician presents the *option* of physician-assisted suicide will be adversely affected by the physician's deep-down belief that the patient should die.

> Insofar as [the differences in power between patient and physician] stem from disparity of education, wealth, and social standing, they will bulk especially large in a doctor's relationship with the poor and the otherwise marginalized. Insofar as they stem from the physician's medical expertise, they will be an especially salient feature of the doctor-patient relationship when the patient is desperately or terminally ill. They therefore pose the danger that any discussion in which the doctor attempts to

determine the genuineness of the patient's willingness and consent will also be one in which what the doctor says and what the doctor concludes about the patient's state of mind will be colored by the doctor's view that the patient would be better off if her life were over. They pose the danger that patients who choose to end their own lives are doing what they believe their doctor wants them to do, rather than acting from a genuine desire of their own.[31]

Robert Burt is even more blunt: "Rules governing doctor-patient relations must not rest on the premise that anyone's wish to help a desperately pained, apparently helpless person is intertwined with a wish to hurt that person, to obliterate him from sight."[32]

The concern is the danger that a patient with a serious illness will not seek medical treatment because of the fear of the conflict of interest between the physician's duties of doing good and not harm, and the physician's desire to hasten the patient's death. A patient whose physician actively educates about the availability of physician-assisted suicide may believe the physician to be more concerned about costs than the patient's human dignity.

Patients at the end of life frequently experience emotional, social, and spiritual suffering. Remember, suffering that is emotional or spiritual in nature may *also* be intolerable. Terminally ill patients also suffer from undiagnosed and untreated clinical depression. Clinical depression not only harms the patient's quality of life but patients with affective disorders die earlier. Clinical depression is strongly correlated with shorter survival.[33]

The symptoms of depression, such as fatigue, loss of appetite, and sleep disturbances mimic symptoms experienced by terminally ill patients. As a result, affective disorders frequently are undiagnosed and untreated in the terminally ill. The argument here goes that even *diagnosed clinical depression* may go untreated, simply because the patient "is going to die anyway." Clinical depression causes anhedonia, increased pain and increased inability to cope with it, anxiety, withdrawal and loss of connection with loved ones, loss of meaning, and an inability to bring forgiveness and the resolution of issues in relationships, bringing them current and closed.

Concerns have been expressed because the California End of Life Option Act provides that depression that does not affect a patient's decision-making capacity is not a bar to receiving a prescription for lethal medication. Not Dead Yet argues that psychologists and psychiatrists are not immune to prejudice against the disabled: "In some cases, they are just as likely as anyone to say, 'If I were in your shoes, I might want to die,' and render an opinion that treatment for depression is not necessary, paving the way for a lethal solution."[34]

Evaluating Requests for Hastened Death

Taking a large step back now from that rich ground of moral argument, we can observe that many patients who are afraid of future suffering ask their physicians about hastened death. Many patients will not use the prescription but may nonetheless be comforted by the *availability* of the lethal medication—it's mere existence gives them a vital reassurance of some measure of personal control, over *something*. Other patients will be demanding immediate help, right this second.

In either case, a patient's request must never be dismissed. The physician needs to be open to a respectful discussion, to assisting the patient "to think out loud." To dismiss a request off-hand is to shut the patient up, to close the door to communication, and is effectively abandoning him or her. Patients are profoundly comforted by the willingness of their physicians to hear their concerns and to take them seriously. "It is a rare patient with a life-threatening illness who doesn't think about suicide, if only in passing."[35]

Case 15-2. The Supreme Court Amici Briefs.

The following are excerpts from affidavits of patients asking for physician-assisted suicide that were attached to amici briefs filed with the Supreme Court in Washington v Glucksberg and Vacco v Quill. As you read them, think about why these patients requested physician-assisted suicide. Consider carefully with each case what it really means to "die with dignity."

Patient A is a sixty-nine-year-old retired pediatrician who has suffered since 1988 from cancer that has now metastasized throughout her skeleton. Although she tried and benefitted temporarily from various treatments including chemotherapy and radiation, she is now in the terminal phase of her disease. In November of 1993, her doctor referred her to hospice care. Only patients with a life expectancy of less than six months are eligible for such care. Patient A has been almost completely bedridden since June of 1993 and experiences constant pain, which becomes especially sharp and severe when she moves. The only treatment available to her at this time is medication, which cannot fully alleviate her pain. In addition, she suffers from swollen legs, bed sores, poor appetite, nausea and vomiting, impaired vision, incontinence of bowel, and general weakness. Patient A is mentally competent and wishes to formally hasten her death by taking prescribed drugs.

Patient B, a seventy-six-year-old retired physical education instructor who was dying of thyroid cancer stated:

I have a large cancerous tumor which is wrapped around the right carotid artery in my neck and is collapsing my esophagus and invading my voice box. The tumor has significantly reduced my ability to swallow and prevents me from eating anything but very thin liquids in extremely small amounts. The cancer has metastasized to my pleural cavity and it is painful to yawn or cough. In early July 1994, I had a feeding tube implanted and have suffered serious problems as a result. I take a variety of medications to manage the pain. It is not possible for me to reduce my pain to an acceptable or comfortable level and to retain an alert state. At this time, it is clear to me, based on the advice of my doctors, that I am in the terminal phase of this disease. At the point at which I can no longer endure the pain and suffering associated with my cancer, I want to have drugs available for the purpose of hastening my death in a humane and certain manner. I want to be able to discuss freely with my treating physician my intention of hastening my death through the consumption of drugs prescribed for that purpose.

Patient C is a forty-four-year-old artist dying of AIDS. Since his diagnosis in 1991, he has experienced two bouts of pneumonia, chronic severe skin and sinus infections, grand mal seizures and extreme fatigue. He has already lost 70% of his vision to cytomegalovirus retinitis, a degenerative disease which will result in blindness and rob him of his ability to paint. His doctor has indicated that he is in the terminal phase of his illness. Patient C is especially cognizant of the suffering imposed by a lingering terminal illness because he was the primary caregiver for his long-term companion who died of AIDS in June of 1991. He also observed his grandfather's death from diabetes preceded by multiple amputations as well as loss of vision and hearing. Patient C is mentally competent, and understands there is no cure for AIDS. He has asked his physician for drugs to hasten his inevitable death after enduring four excruciatingly painful months because he did not wish to die in a hospital in a drug-induced stupor.

Patient D stated:

> My illness began with my stomach and colon. I had severe diarrhea, fevers and wasting. In February 1994, I was diagnosed with microsporidiosis, a parasitic infection for which there is effectively no treatment. At approximately the same time, I contracted AIDS-related pneumonia. The pneumonia's infusion therapy treatment was so extremely toxic that I vomited with each infusion. In March 1994, I was diagnosed with cryptosporidiosis, a parasitic infection which has caused severe diarrhea–sometimes producing twenty stools a day–extreme abdominal pain, nausea and additional significant wasting. I have begun to lose bowel control. For each of these conditions I have undergone a variety of medical treatments, each of which has had significant adverse side effects. While I have tolerated some nightly intravenous feedings, I am unwilling to accept this for an extended period of time. I understand that there are no cures. I can no longer endure the pain and suffering, and I want to have drugs available for the purpose of hastening my death.

Patient E is a sixty-nine-year-old retired sales representative who suffers from emphysema, which causes him a constant sensation of suffocating. He is connected to an oxygen tank at all times and takes morphine regularly to calm the panic reaction associated with his feeling of suffocation. Patient E also suffers from heart failure related to his pulmonary disease which obstructs the flow of blood to his extremities and causes severe leg pain. There are no cures for his pulmonary and cardiac conditions and he is in the terminal phase of his illness. [Later, Patient E is mentally competent and wishes to commit suicide by taking physician-prescribed drugs. Patient E's physician refused his request because he feared prosecution. Denied medical assistance, Patient E ended his life by jumping from the West Seattle Bridge and plummeting to his death. Fortunately, he did not survive the plunge and require permanent hospitalization in an even more exacerbated state of pain.]

Patient G, a forty-eight-year-old publishing executive suffering from AIDS, stated:

> At this time I have almost no immune system function. My first major illness associated with AIDS was cryptosporidiosis, a parasitic infection which caused me severe fevers and diarrhea and associated pain, suffering and exhaustion. I also suffer from cytomegalovirus retinitis. An AIDS-related virus which attacks the retina and causes blindness. To date I have become almost completely blind in my left eye. I am at risk of losing my sight altogether from this condition. I also suffer from toxoplasmosis, a parasitic infection which has caused lesions to develop on my brain. I take daily infusions of cytovene for the retinitis condition. This medication, administered for an hour through a Hickman tube which is connected to an artery in my chest, prevents me from ever taking showers and makes simple routine functions burdensome. In addition, I inject my leg daily with neupogen to combat the deficient white cell count in my blood. The daily injection of this medication is extremely painful. At this point it is clear to me, based on the advice of my doctors, that I am in the terminal phase of AIDS. It is my desire that my physician prescribe suitable drugs for me to consume for the purpose of hastening my death when and if my suffering becomes intolerable.

191

Patient H, like many terminally ill patients, killed himself in a secretive and lonely fashion, in order to spare his family from possible criminal charges. As a result, he was deprived of a chance to die in a dignified manner with his loved ones at his side. The man's daughter described her father's death this way:

> When he realized that my family was going to be away for a day, he wrote us a beautiful letter, went down to his basement and shot himself with his 12-gauge shotgun. He was 84. My son-in-law then had the unfortunate and unpleasant task of cleaning my father's splattered brains off the basement walls.

Case 15-3. The Case of David Rivlin.

The case of David Rivlin, superficially about the withdrawal of life-sustaining treatment, is really about the minimal value that we place on the lives of disabled persons. David, as a result of an accident at age twenty, was intellectually unimpaired, but so severely paralyzed that he depended on a ventilator to breathe. He lay in a bed in a skilled nursing facility staring out the window at a brick wall. The Detroit Free Press wrote: "[N]othing. . . could tune out the sound that symbolized his ultimate imprisonment: the incessant whir of a respirator sitting on a chipped wooden night stand close enough to allow its hose to reach through the hole in his throat." People magazine also interviewed him. He said, "The respirator takes away all choice in your life ... I don't want to live an empty life lying helplessly in a nursing home another thirty years."

In 1989, David decided that he wanted to die, and petitioned a court to order his physicians to disconnect his ventilator. The judge agreed, reasoning that withdrawing the ventilator would not be physician-assisted suicide, and therefore illegal at the time. The judge gave David the order because he rightly reasoned that this was a case of David's refusing medical treatment and he had this right. David's physician turned off the ventilator and he died almost immediately.

In the 1970's, David had been unable to get enough money from Michigan Social Services so that he might live independently with paid caregivers. In 1981, the Michigan rules changed, and David could have received more money. David did not know and no social worker had applied for money for him under the new rule. When the articles in The Detroit Free Press and People appeared, quadriplegics wrote him letters encouraging him to live. The nursing facility staff did not take the time to read him the letters.

Ostensibly, this is a case about the withdrawal of life-sustaining treatment. But really it is a case about quality of life and the lived experience of many persons with disabilities without social and human support. Had David not been dependent on a ventilator which could be withdrawn, he might not have requested hastened death, either physician-assisted suicide or euthanasia.[36]

Bioethicist Howard Brody, who had supported David's request to remove the ventilator, later wrote:

> I am now embarrassed to realize how limited was the basis on which I made my decisions about David Rivlin. . . [T]here was no medical need for Rivlin to be effectively incarcerated in a nursing home. If Rivlin had been given access to a reasonable amount of community resources, of the sort that other persons with disabilities were making use of at the time, he could have been moved out of the nursing home and probably could have had his

own apartment. He could have been much more able to see friends, get outside a bit, and generally have a much more interesting and stimulating life. . .. If we look at a case one way, it seems that the problem is the person's physical disability. If we shift our view, we realize that the problem is not the disability, but rather the refusal of society to make reasonable and not terribly expensive accommodations to it. . . This is the key lesson that disabilities advocates are trying to teach the rest of us. . . There's every reason to believe in hindsight that David Rivlin died unnecessarily, and that we who claimed to care about his "rights" should have been demanding that services be made available for him rather than that he be allowed to die.[37]

Conclusion

There is a very fundamental difference between mercy and compassion.

Compassion is an awareness of suffering, at best empathy—at worse, a vague sentiment of sympathy. Mercy is an action to alleviate the suffering of one who is powerless and under our direct control. It is all fine and good to have compassion for the patient, but unless we admit that the patient's suffering is under our control, we will never be able to have real mercy. To have mercy is to *act*. To have compassion is to *feel*. Compassion without mercy can be paralyzing.

Most of us are not taught to do anything better than to control, to treat, and to fight for a cure. But, when the chances of the cure are so remote as to be meaningless, compassion is no longer enough. We must have mercy for those patients who are entrapped in technology, are reflexively treated, and who cannot speak for themselves. As healthcare providers, we do things to patients that we would not want done to us, *all the time*. We do not see it because we do not want to look. Because of what, in looking, it would say about ourselves.

If death is inevitable (or even highly likely) good palliative care, including palliative sedation and hospice, can be merciful. If we use our options for mercy, then we do not need to go so far as mercy killing. However, if we remain a culture that either fights or ignores the inevitability of death and if we continue to treat without reflection, then mercy will inevitably end in mercy killing—because patients will be afraid that they will never be allowed to die otherwise. The core ethos of the medical establishment, to treat and treat again, will drive us to end our suffering by ending ourselves.

Mercy does not always mean action. Sometimes, it can mean bearing witness to suffering without acting in any way, and by being silent. The capacity for presence will stop us from trying to convert the patient's goals to our agenda. For the first few weeks when I first started working in medical centers, I wanted to do something, *anything*, to save myself from having to be present to and witness suffering. I quickly learned that silence and presence can be merciful. And I learned that the act of presence can change the one who is present in many ways.

Over a decade of teaching students lies behind this book. I can tell how unfamiliar is the concept of letting a life go, and how reluctant students are to acknowledge that there is another way. They cannot think it possible because they have never been taught that it is possible. But soon, their intuition for mercy finds freedom and they know how to act in a healthcare culture that is relentless and out of control. I have hope. And I hope that this book can bring you hope as well.

Index

202

204

205

REFERENCES

Chapter 1: Quality of Life

[1] Thomas A. Shannon and James J. Walter, "The PVS Patient and Forgoing/Withdrawing Medical Nutrition and Hydration," *Theological Studies* 49 (December, 1988): 623-647.

[2] Ibid.

[3] Ibid.

[4] Edward W. Keyserlink, "The Quality of Life and Death," in Secretary of the Law Reform Commission of Canada, *Sanctity of Life or Quality of Life in the Context of Ethics, Medicine and Law*, reprinted in *Quality of Life: The New Medical Dilemma*, eds. James J. Walter and Thomas A. Shannon (New York and Mahwah, N.J., 1990)

Chapter 2: Killing vs. Allowing to Die

[1] Cruzan v. Director, Missouri Department of Health, 497 U.S. 261 (1990), was the first "right to die" case decided by the United States Supreme Court. Nancy Cruzan was a patient in a persistent vegetative state whose biological life was sustained by a gastrostomy tube delivering artificial nutrition and hydration directly into her stomach. The Court affirmed the earlier ruling of the Supreme Court of Missouri, ruling that the State of Missouri could require "clear and convincing evidence" of a patient's wishes for withdrawal of life-sustaining treatment. Clear and convincing evidence of Nancy's wishes were discovered, and she was allowed to die. The Court also discussed the importance of advance directives.

[2] Michael D. Bayles, "Euthanasia and the Quality of Life," in *Medical Treatment of the Dying: Moral Issues*, eds. Michael D. Bayles and Dallas M. High (Rochester, VT: Schenkman Books, 1978).

[3] Ibid.

[4] Institute of Medicine, Committee on Care at the End of Life, *Approaching Death: Improving Care at the End of Life* (Washington DC: National Academy Press, 1997) 14.

[5] President's Commission for the Study of Ethical Problems in Medicine and Biomedical and Behavioral Research, *Deciding to Forego Life-Sustaining Treatment: A Report on the Ethical, Medical, and Legal Issues in Treatment Decisions* (Washington DC: U.S. Government Printing Office, 1983: 81.

[6] "There is no ethical distinction between withdrawing and withholding life-sustaining treatment." Council on Ethical and Judicial Affairs, American Medical Association, "5.3 Withholding or Withdrawing Life-Sustaining Treatment," *AMA Code of Medical Ethics* (2016), https://www.ama-ssn.org/sites/default/files/media-browser/code-of-medical-ethics-chapter-5.pdf, accessed May 11, 2017. Several justices of the United States Supreme Court also have ruled that there is no legal distinction between withholding treatment and withdrawing treatment. See Cruzan v. Director 497 U.S. 261 (1990) (the withdrawal of artificial nutrition and hydration from a persistent vegetative state patient); see also Washington v. Glucksberg 521 U.S. 702 (1997), and Vacco v. Quill 521 U.S. 793 (1997).

[7] Faber-Langendoen, Kathy M.D. and Paul Lanken, M.D., "Dying Patients in the Intensive Care Unit: Forgoing Treatment, Maintaining Care," developed for the ACP–ASIM End-of-Life Care Consensus Panel (2000), *Annals of Internal Medicine* (December 2000): 886-93.

Chapter 3: Ordinary and Extraordinary Treatment

[1] President's Commission, 88.

[2] Shannon and Walter.

[3] American Medical Association Position Statement on End of Life Care and Advance Care Planning, https://ama.com.au/system/tdf/documents/AMA_position_statement_on_end_of_life_care_and_advance_care_planning_2014.pdf?file=1&type=node&id=40573, accessed July 14, 2017.

[4] President's Commission, 86-87.

[5] Shannon and Walter.

1

[2] Pope John Paul II, "Address of John Paul II to the Participants in the International Congress on Life-Sustaining Treatments and Vegetative State: Scientific Advances and Ethics Dilemmas" (Rome: The Holy See, March 20, 2014), http://w2.vatican.va/content/john-paul-ii/en/speeches/2004/march/documents/hf_jp-ii_spe_20040320_congress-fiamc.html, accessed May 11, 2017.

[3] Michael Panicola, "Catholic Teaching on Prolonging Life," *The Hastings Center Report* (Nov/Dec 2001):31,6.

[4] Ibid.

[5]Position of the American Academy of Neurology on certain aspects of the care and management of the persistent vegetative state patient. Adopted by the Executive Board, American Academy of Neurology, *Neurology* 39(1) (January 1, 1989): 125-126.

[6]Robert L. Fine, M.D., "From Quinlan to Schiavo: medical, ethical, and legal issues in severe brain injury," *Proc(Bayl). Univ. Med. Centr)*. 14(4) (October, 2005).

The Multi-Society Task Force on PVS, "Medical Aspects of the Persistent Vegetative State," *New England Journal of Medicine* 330(1) (June 2, 1994), converted to 2013 dollars according to the Centers for Medicare and Medicaid, Services, index in health care costs, https://www.cms.gov/Research-Statistics-Data-and-Systems/Statistics-Trends-and-Reports/NationalHealthExpendData/Downloads/HistoricalNHEPaper.pdf (accessed March 16, 2017).

[7] Stuart J Younger, M.D., quoted in "Commentary: Getting Rational about Health-care Rationing: The right-to-die debate sidesteps the real issue: A need to reapportion care," *Bloomberg Business Week*, November 16, 2003 9:00 PM PST).

[8] Eric Racine, PhD, et al, "Media coverage of the persistent vegetative state and end-of-life decision-making, *Neurology* 71(13) (Sep 23, 2008).

[9] Lindsay A. Hampson and Ezekiel J. Emanuel, "The Prognosis for Changes in End-Of-Life Care After the Schiavo Case, *Health Affairs* 24(4) (2005).

[10] Gary Langer, "Poll: No Role for Government in Schiavo Case," *ABC News*, March 21, 2005. http://abcnews.go.com/Politics/PollVault/story?id=599622.

[11] Conservatorship of the Person of Robert Wendland, 26 Cal. 4th 522 (2001).

[12] Amici Curiae Brief of Not Dead Yet, et al, filed in Wendland.

[13] Alzheimer's Association Position Statement, "Assisted Oral Feeding and Tube Feeding." accessed March 17, 2017.

[14] Ibid.

[15] American Geriatrics Society Ethics Committee and Clinical Practice and Models of Care Committee, American Geriatrics Society Position Statement, "Feeding tubes in advanced dementia position statement," *Journal of the American Geriatric Society*, 62(8) (August, 2014). "When Evidence Clashes with Emotion: Feeding Tubes in Advanced Dementia," *Annals of Long-Term Care: Clinical Care and Aging* 22(9) (2014): 24-26.

[16] Ibid.

[17] Sam Savage, "Starvation is Not Painful, Experts Say," quoting Ira Byock, MD, in Red Orbit (March 24, 2005), http://www.redorbit.com/news/health/138158/starvation_is_not_painful_experts_say/ (accessed July 14, 2017).

Chapter 5: Informed Consent

[1] *Pater* means "father" in Latin.

[2] Council on Ethical and Judicial Affairs of the American Medical Association, "Opinion 8.08 - Informed Choice," *Current Opinions with Annotations* (2012-2013 edition).

[3] AMA Opinion 8.08.

Chapter 6: Decision-Making Capacity

[1] *See* California Probate Code Section 4657. (Added by Stats. 1999, Ch. 658, Sec. 39. Effective January 1, 2000. Operative July 1, 2000, by Sec. 43 of Ch. 658.).

[2] Allen E. Buchanan and Dan W. Brock, *Deciding for Others: The Ethics of Surrogate Decision Making* (Cambridge: Cambridge University Press (1990), 18.

[3] Ibid., 25.

[4] Ibid. 26, 28.

[5] Ibid., 84.

[6] Ibid., 85.

[7] Ibid., 49-50.

[8] Ibid., 50-51.

[9] Ibid., 83.

[10] Ibid., 52.

[11] Ibid., 85.

[12] Marc Tunzi, "Can the Patient Decide? Evaluating Patient Capacity in Practice," *American Physician* 64(2) (July 15, 2001): 299-308.

[13] Ibid.

[14] Ibid.

[15]Buchanan and Brock, 72.

[16] Ibid., 73.

Chapter 7: Decision-Making for Incapacitated Patients

[1] *See* California Probate Code Section 4643.

[2] Cruzan v. Director.

[3] Council on Ethical and Judicial Affairs of the American Medical Association, "Opinion 2-20 – Withholding or Withdrawing Life-Sustaining Medical Treatment," *Code of Medical Ethics* (2012-2013).

[4] The common law hearsay rule in legal cases states that testimony or documents which speak about persons who are not in the court are not admissible into evidence. The first-hand witness, the person who supposedly knew the facts, is not in court to state his exact words, the judge or the jury cannot judge his demeanor and credibility, and the other party's lawyer cannot cross-examine him, i.e., ask questions. There are many exceptions to the hearsay rule which are not applicable here.

[5] Annette Rid and David Wendler, "Use of a Patient Preference Predictor to Help Make Medical Decisions for Incapacitated Patients," *The Journal of Medicine and Philosophy* 39(2) (April, 2014): 104-129.

[6] President's Commission for the Study of Ethical Problems in Medicine and Biomedical and Behavioral Research, 135.

[7] Ibid. 185.

Chapter 8: Advance Directives and Physician Orders for Life-Sustaining Treatment (POLST)

[1] Colby, William H., *Unplugged: Reclaiming Our Right to Die in America* (New York: AMACON (2006), 141.

[2] Steven B. Hardin, M.D. and Yasmin A. Yusufaly, M.D., "Difficult end-of-life treatment decisions: do other factors trump advance directives?" *Archives of Internal Medicine* 164(14) (July 26, 2004). (A survey revealed that 65 percent of physicians said they would not follow an advance directive if the instructions conflicted with the physician's own opinions about the patient's prognosis or expected quality of life).

Chapter 9: Futility

[1] Edward Pellegrino. "Decisions at the end of life — the abuse of the concept of futility," *Practical Bioethics* 1(3) (2005): 3-6.

[2] Institute of Medicine, 127

[3] Task Force on Ethics of the Society of Critical Care Medicine, "Consensus report on the ethics of foregoing life-sustaining treatments in the critically ill." *Critical Care Medicine* 18(2) (December, 1990).

[4] Elizabeth B. Lamont and Nicholas A. Christakis, "Prognostic Disclosure to Patients with Cancer Near the End of Life," *Annals of Internal Medicine* 134(2) (June 19, 2001). Sandra H. Johnson, "Making Room for Dying: End of Life Care in Nursing Homes," *Hastings Center Report* (November/December, 2005). Cited in Colby, 111.

[5] David Crippen, "Commentary: Medical treatment for the terminally ill; 'the risk of unacceptable badness'." *Critical Care* (19) (published online May 10, 2005). accessed March 17, 2017.

[6] Lawrence J. Schneiderman, M.D., "Defining Medical Futility and Improving Medical Care." *Journal of Bioethical Inquiry* 8(2) (June, 2011): 123–131.

[7] Lawrence J. Schneiderman, M.D., *et al.*, "Medical Futility: Its Meaning and Ethical Implications," *Annals of Internal Medicine* 112(12) (June 15, 1990): 949-54.

[8] Ibid.

[9] Schneiderman, "Defining Medical Futility."

[10] President's Commission for the Study of Ethical Problems in Medicine and Biomedical and Behavioral Research, 190

[11] President's Commission for the Study of Ethical Problems in Medicine and Biomedical and Behavioral Research, 191

[12] See Cruzan vs. Director.

[13] Institute of Medicine, 15

[14] Council on Ethical and Judicial Affairs, American Medical Association, "Guidelines for the Appropriate Use of Do-Not-Resuscitate Orders," *Journal of the American Medical Association* 265(14) (April 10, 1990): 1868-71.

[15] Colby, 116, citing Kaufman, Sharon, *And a Time to Die: How American Hospitals Shape the End of Life* (New York: Scribner, 2005), 49.

[16] President's Commission for the Study of Ethical Problems in Medicine and Biomedical and Behavioral Research, 234.

[17] President's Commission for the Study of Ethical Problems in Medicine and Biomedical and Behavioral Research, 247

[18] President's Commission for the Study of Ethical Problems in Medicine and Biomedical and Behavioral Research, 249.

[19] President's Commission for the Study of Ethical Problems in Medicine and Biomedical and Behavioral Research, 250-251

[20] Uniform Health-Care Decisions Act [24-7A-1 NMSA 1978] *See also,* Council on Ethical and Judicial Affairs of the American Medical Association, "Opinion 2.037 Medical futility in end-of-life care." *Code of Medical Ethics*. Medical center futility policies will be discussed in the chapter on ethics committees.

[21] David Barnard, Institute to Enhance Palliative Care, Palliative Care Case of the Month, "The family that doesn't get it.'" (September, 2005). accessed March 17, 2017.

[22] Ibid.

[23] Ibid.

[24] Ibid.

[25] *See, for example*, Braden J. Manns, *et al.*, "An economic evaluation of activated protein C treatment for severe sepsis," N*ew England Journal of Medicine* 347(13) (September 26, 2002).

[26] Judith E Nelson, et al., "Chronic Critical Illness," American Journal of Respiratory and Critical Care Medicine 182(4) (August 15, 2010): 446–454.; Christopher E Cox, "An Economic Evaluation of Prolonged Mechanical Ventilation," Critical Care Medicine 35(8) (August, 2007).

[27] Nelson, et al.

[28] Nelson, et al.

Chapter 10: Healthcare Allocation

[29] Nelson, et al.

[30] Nelson, et al.

[31] Nelson, et al.

[1] World Bank Health Expenditure, Total (% of GDP). http://data.worldbank.org/indicator/SH.XPD.TOTL.ZS/(accessed May 28, 2017).

[2] United States Food and Drug Administration, "The Impact of Direct-to-Consumer Advertising." https://www.fda.gov/Drugs/ResourcesForYou/Consumers/ucm143562.htm (accessed May 28, 2017).

[3] Keehan, Sean, et a., "National Health Expenditure Projections, 2015–25: Economy, Prices, And Aging Expected to Shape Spending and Enrollment," *Health Affairs*, published ahead of print July 13, 2016 at http://content.healthaffairs.org/content/early/2016/07/12/hlthaff.2016.0459 (accessed May 28, 2017).

[4] *See* David Goodman, M.D., *et al.*, for The Dartmouth Institute for Health Policy and Clinical Practice, "Trends in Cancer Care at the End of Life: A Dartmouth Atlas of Health Care Brief" (September 4, 2013). accessed March 17, 2017.

[5] Colby, 102.

[6] California Health Care Foundation, "Measuring Up? End-of-Life Cancer Care in California," Dartmouth Atlas of Health Care.

[7] Goodman, *et al.,* footnote 2., citing Amber E. Barnato, *et al.,* "Are regional variations in end-of-life care intensity explained by patient preferences? A study of the US Medicare population." *Medical Care* 45(5) (June, 2007).

[8] Ibid.

[9] "Spending in the Last Year of Life and the Impact of Hospice on Medicare Outlays," a report by Direct Research, LLC, for the Medicare Payment Advisory Commission. accessed March 17, 2017.

[10] Elliott Fisher, M.D., *et al.,* "Health Care 2009: Slowing the Growth of Health Care Costs—Lessons from Regional Variation," New England Journal of Medicine 360(9) (February 26, 2009), analyzing the Dartmouth Atlas data.

[11] Intelligence[2] Debate "Ration End of Life Care," statements by Arthur Kellermann. accessed March 17, 2017.

Chapter 12: Palliative Sedation

[1] Timothy Kirk, *et al.,* for the Palliative Sedation Task Force of the National Hospice and Palliative Care Organization Ethics Committee of the National Hospice and Palliative Care Organization (NHPCO), "Position Statement and Commentary on the Use of Palliative Sedation in Imminently Dying Terminally Ill Patients," *Journal of Pain and Symptom Management* 39(5) (May, 2010).

[2] Timothy Quill, M.D. and Ira Byock, M.D., "Responding to Intractable Terminal Suffering: The Role of Terminal Sedation and Voluntary Refusal of Food and Fluids," *Annals of Internal Medicine* 132(5) (March 7, 2000).

[3] Council of Ethical and Judicial Affairs of the American Medical Association, Opinion 2.201 – "Sedation to Unconsciousness in End-of-Life Care, *Code of Medical Ethics* (2012-2013).

[4] National Hospice and Palliative Care Organization (NHPCO).

[5] Quill and Byock.

[6] Ibid.

[7] Christof Muller-Busch, *et al.,* "Sedation in palliative care – a critical analysis of 7 years' experience," *BMC Palliative Care* (published online on May 13, 2003). Accessed May 11, 2017.

[8] Quill and Byock.

[9] Improving Death, 26

214

[10] National Hospice and Palliative Care Organization (NHPCO).

[11] Ibid.

[12] Marco Maltoni, *et al.*, "Palliative sedation therapy does not hasten death: results from a prospective multicenter study." *Annals of Oncology* (20) (August, 2009).:1163-69.

[13] Quill and Byock.

[14] See, Cruzan vs. Director.

[15] Quill and Byock.

[16] Ibid.

[17] Linda Ganzini, M.D., *et al.*, "Nurses' Experiences with Hospice Patients Who Refuse Food and Fluids to Hasten Death," *New England Journal of Medicine* (July 24, 2003). 2003: 359-365.

[18] Quill and Byock.

[19] Ibid.

[20] Ibid.

[21] Ganzini, *et al.*

[22] Quill and Byock.

[23] Ibid.

Chapter 14: The Principle of Double Effect

[1] AMA H-140.966 Decisions Near the End of Life. See also California Assembly Bill 2747. End of Life Care.

[2] *See* James J. Walter, "Proportionate reason and its three levels of inquiry: structuring the ongoing debate," *Proportionalism: For and Against*, Christopher Kaczor, ed. (Milwaukee, Marquette University Press: 2000).

Chapter 15: Physician-Assisted Suicide

[1] Amicus Curiae Brief of Not Dead Yet, et al. in Alberto R. Gonzalez, Attorney General v. Oregon 546 U.S. 243 (2006).

[2] Intelligence[2] Debate, "Legalize Assisted Suicide," statements by Peter Singer, accessed March 17, 2017.

[3] Amicus Curiae Brief of Bioethicists in *Vacco v. Quill* 521 US 793 (1997), and *Washington v. Glucksberg* 521 US 702 (1997).

[4] Quill and Byock.

[5] Ibid.

[6] Antonio Filiberti, *et al.*, "Characteristics of terminal cancer patients who committed suicide during a home palliative care program," *Journal of Pain and Symptom Management* 22(1) (August, 2001):544-53.

[7] Oregon Death with Dignity Act: 2016 Data Summary, Table 1.

[8] Carl Wellman, "A Legal Right to Physician-Assisted Suicide Defended," *Social Theory and Practice* 29(1) (January, 2003): 19-38.

[9] Quill and Byock.

[10] Ibid.

[11] Timothy Quill, M.D., "Death and dignity. A case of individualized decision making," *New England Journal of Medicine* 324(1) (March 7, 1991).

[12] Anthony L. Bach, M.D., *et al.*, "Physician Assisted Suicide and Euthanasia in Washington State," *Journal of the American Medical Association* 275(12) (March 27, 1996): 919-25.

[13] Gallup, "In U.S., Support Up for Doctor-Assisted Suicide." (May 27, 2015). Accessed March 27, 2017.

[14] Amicus Curiae Brief of Bioethicists.

[15] Susan Okie, "Country's Doctors Remain Divided Over Physician-Assisted Suicide," *Washington Post* (January 8, 1997). accessed March 17, 2017.

[16] Council on Ethical and Religious Affairs of the American Medical Association "Opinion 2.211 - Physician-Assisted Suicide," *Code of Medical Ethics* 2012-1013.

[17] California Medical Association Press Release "California Medical Association removes opposition to physician aid in dying bill" (May 20, 2015).

[18] Council on Ethical and Judicial Affairs, "Opinion 2.211 - Physician-Assisted Suicide."

[19] American Medical Association Resolution, "H-140.966 Decisions Near the End of Life." accessed March 17, 2017.

[20] National Hospice & Palliative Care Organization (NHPCO), "Commentary and Resolution on Physician Assisted Suicide." accessed March 17, 2017.

[21] Adrienne Asch, "Recognizing Death while Affirming Life: Can End of Life Reform Uphold a Disabled Person's Interest in Continued Life?" in *Improving End of Life Care: Why Has It Been So Difficult? Hastings Center Report Special Report* (November-December 2005): S31-S36.

[22] Ibid.

[23] U.S. Congress. House. Testimony of Diane Coleman, president of Not Dead Yet of Forest Park. Illinois, before the Subcommittee on Criminal Justice, Drug Policy and Human Resources of the Committee on Government Reform of the U.S. House of Representatives (April 19, 2005).

[24] U.S. Congress. Senate. Testimony of Diane Coleman, president of Not Dead Yet of Forest Park, Illinois, before the United States Senate Judiciary Subcommittee on the Constitution, Civil Rights and Property Rights by Diane Coleman, president of Not Dead Yet (May 25, 2006).

[25] Amicus Curiae Brief of Not Dead Yet in *Gonzalez v Oregon*.

[26] Not Dead Yet to California Governor Jerry Brown Urging Veto of Assisted Suicide Bill (September 22, 2015). accessed May 11, 2017.

[27] Amicus Curiae Brief of Not Dead Yet in Gonzalez v Oregon.

[28] Paul J. Weithman, "Of Assisted Suicide and 'The Philosophers' Brief'," *Ethics* 109(3) (April, 1999): 548-78.

[29] Institute of Medicine (U.S.) Committee on Advancing Pain Research, Care, and Education, "Disparities in Prevalence and Care in Selected Populations," *Relieving Pain in America: A Blueprint for Transforming Prevention, Care, Education, and Research.* (Washington D.C.: National Academies Press 2011), 2.

[30] Not Dead Yet's letter to Governor Jerry Brown.

[31] Weithman, 559-560.

[32] Asch.

[33] Martine Meyer, M.D., *et al.,* "Depressive symptoms in advanced cancer. Part 2. Depression over time; The role of the palliative care professional," *Journal of Palliative Medicine* 17(7) (October, 2003):604-7.

[34] Not Dead Yet's letter to Governor Jerry Brown.

[35] "Education in Palliative and End-of-life Care – Oncology Participant's Handbook Module 14 Physician-Assisted Suicide,"

http://endlink.lurie.northwestern.edu/physician_assisted_suicide_debate/why.cfm (accessed July 14, 2017).

[36] *See* Margot Dougherty and Sandra Rubin Tessler, "Tiring of Life Without Freedom, Quadriplegic David Rivlin Chooses to Die Among Friends," *People* (August 7, 1989).

[37] Howard Brody, "A bioethicist offers an apology," *Lansing City News* (October 6, 2004).

Made in the USA
Las Vegas, NV
30 June 2021